T0129184

How to Please a Woman In & Out of Bed

2ND EDITION

DAYLLE DEANNA SCHWARTZ

Adams Media

New York   London   Toronto   Sydney   New Delhi

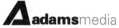

Adams Media
An Imprint of Simon & Schuster, Inc.
57 Littlefield Street
Avon, Massachusetts 02322

For information about special discounts for bulk purchases, please contact Simon & Schuster Special Sales at 1-866-506-1949 or business@simonandschuster.com.

The Simon & Schuster Speakers Bureau can bring authors to your live event. For more information or to book an event contact the Simon & Schuster Speakers Bureau at 1-866-248-3049 or visit our website at www.simonspeakers.com.

Manufactured in the United States of America

Library of Congress Cataloging-in-Publication Data
Schwartz, Daylle Deanna.
How to please a woman in & out of bed / Daylle Deanna Schwartz.—2nd ed.
p.   cm.
ISBN 1-59337-290-6
1. Sex instruction for men. 2. Women—Sexual behavior. 3. Women—Psychology.
4. Man-woman relationships. I. Title: How to please a woman in and out of bed.
II. Title.

HQ36.S38 2005
613.9'6—dc22

                              2004026944

ISBN 978-1-59337-290-3

CONTENTS

Acknowledgments

As always, I must begin by thanking God and the Universe for all of my blessings. Without my strong belief in a higher power, I wouldn't be where I am today!

Thank you to all the men who've taken my workshops or done individual counseling with me and encouraged and inspired me to write this book. Working with you has been a pleasure! A special thank you to all the men and women who contributed knowledge, feelings, and encouragement to my readers through interviews and questionnaires. I sincerely appreciate your taking the time to share your thoughts. It's because of you that the book has so much dimension and spirit.

Thank you again Linda Konner, my terrific agent, for your belief in me and your supportive work on my behalf. Thanks also to Danielle Chiotti, Acquisitions Editor at Adams Media, for being a pleasure to work with. Thank you to Bridget Brace, development editor, for your sharp insight.

BIG, BIG thanks to my wonderfully supportive family. Thanks to my friends who have supported me through my growing pains and my education about men. Thank you Julie Coulter, for sharing so much of yourself and for your always-cheerful encouragement. Thank you Lydia Stein for encouraging me to write this book and your continued support. Thank you Grace Gallo, for always cheering me on. Thank you Judy Wong, for your consistent belief in me and for always being there for the big stuff.

A special thanks to everyone at The Silver Spoon diner on First Avenue in New York City—where I regularly take my laptop out for a yummy meal with terrific service and lots of refills on my coffee. Thanks to some of my ex's for showing me why this book was necessary!

Chapters 13 and 14 are dedicated to the memory of Bay DeLussa, who passed away as I wrote this book. Bay was known to many men for his determination to educate anyone who'd listen about how to satisfy a woman. He saved many marriages by teaching men skills and attitude. I interviewed his son, Jesse DeLussa, who shared many of the techniques that his father advocated. Thank you Jesse for giving me so much time and great info!

Introduction

Men avoid self-help books and classes like the plague and for good reasons:

+ Personal growth is considered a "woman thing"—you want to keep your masculinity intact

+ Women push you to read self-help books—you don't like being told what to do

+ You know that you're different from women—you assume what works for us won't work for you.

I agree. You may be skeptical about reading what I, a woman, tell you about pleasing my own sex. I don't blame you. So—I'll tell you straight up-front that I love you guys, I'm grateful you exist, and I respect your differences from women and don't propose to change your basic essence. It's delicious as is!

I always wanted to write a book for men but was told, "Men don't buy self-help books." Self-help has been looked upon as a woman's thing. But when I taught my "Nice Girls on Top" class, I was regularly asked by men to do one geared to their needs. I began one for men in 1993, which evolved into my Guybercize™ workshops. Men especially enjoy the camaraderie that ensues when they share their frustrations with women. Participants leave the class with their eyes opened wider, as if someone just turned on a light. They show more gratitude than women, who have lots of avenues for gathering understanding. I also do counseling with men, and must admit I enjoy them the most. Men encouraged me to write this book.

I proved the naysayers wrong! You do want to enlighten yourselves and I'm pleased for you. The first edition of *How to Please a Woman In & Out of Bed* has sold so well that I was asked to revise it. In this new edition, I've added sexier tips and more ways to make you appealing to women that shouldn't be uncomfortable. I know that women can be difficult to decipher and seem even more difficult to please. They get on my nerves too! I often prefer the company of men because of that. But since you want to be in our company, and our beds, read on.

Why do men and women often seem so incompatible? Think of relationships in terms of computers. As kids, our hard drives are programmed differently. Women are more like Macs. Men are more like PCs. Macs have always been able to read PCs better than PCs could read Macs. Men often have no clue about what women are trying to say. Women analyze you until they find a conclusion, however wrong it is. Macs are considered to be more creative, and women go into more nuances and details than many of you think necessary. But, with the right software we can be compatible. Look how much better PCs can now read Macs since Bill Gates designed better software. Consider this book YOUR software!

I respect your right to be men—your right to be different from us, your right to have your idiosyncrasies just as we do, and your right not to follow standards that we dictate. I believe you can get along with women better, without feeling you have to sell yourself to our whims.

Do you find the concept of self-help uncomfortable (if not worse)? I've developed tech support just for you! My approach will empower you by providing tools for solving problems in your interaction with women. Instead of a traditional self-help approach, I'll teach you techniques from my workshops and help you stretch the boundaries of the stereotypical upbringing that programs many guys. More flexibility allows a new approach to dealing with us women. By opening yourself up to a revised way of understanding our gender, you'll own the power to enjoy a much happier and more relaxed relationship with your lady, and probably have more great sex! How could that be bad?

When I wrote my book *All Men Are Jerks Until Proven Otherwise*, men regularly asked for a peek at the manuscript. I incorrectly assumed they wanted to see if I was male bashing. (For the record, I wasn't.) They were actually looking for clues to understanding women. Some thought that reading my advice would give them an idea about how to please us.

What do women want? You ask me this all the time, as you increasingly find us harder to understand. The truth is, women themselves are still trying to figure out what they want. Many of us don't quite have a grip on how to handle and grow with the increasing freedom being given to us. How can we tell you what we want if we don't know the answer ourselves? We may know what we'd ideally like, but are scared to buck the system and ask for it. Our reactions to inner conflicts can drive you guys nuts. Why shouldn't they? They drive us nuts too!

Becoming an individual is confusing for many women, me included. We want independence, yet still depend on you for a lot of our happiness. We want to be assertive and confident, yet we get messages from you that it's unfeminine. We want to be your equals, but often don't know how. We say we don't want special treatment, yet we do need to feel special. Guys, we're having a tough time getting comfortable with ourselves! Please bear with us!

Our original programs—the messages we got growing up—taught many of us that we need a man to be complete, so we expect you to fill every need and be our main source of happiness. Many of us can't let go of old "rules," even when we want to, just like many of you. So we confuse the heck out of those of you who'd sincerely like to understand our needs, since we don't always understand them either. What a dilemma!

Do you feel as though you're fighting a battle against women with no weapons? We arm ourselves as you retreat, absorbing knowledge from self-help books and classes faster than you can turn your back on them. Then we drive you crazy with demands and rules. Instead of solving problems, the personal growth of women can create more, because a greater imbalance develops between the sexes. As we work on self-improvement, many of you complain that women can be demanding, sometimes irrational creatures.

Do you deal with problems by hoping they'll go away on their own? Sweeties, that's a short-term fix which makes them worse in the long run! You may need help but aren't comfortable getting it. Maybe you were raised to handle things yourself, or your ego pushes you to simply grit your teeth and tolerate our shticks. Or, you've given up.

So you struggle without a clue about how to please us as we expect more from you. That's why you should continue reading.

I do believe men and women can live together in peace, and even harmony. We can learn to thoroughly enjoy pleasuring each other in bed to an extent most of you think exists only in fantasy. It takes effort and communication from both partners. It takes understanding and respecting each other's needs. If you keep waiting for *her* to learn a magic technique to change into your dream woman, sit down. You don't want to be standing while you wait the rest of your life.

The second edition of *How to Please a Woman In & Out of Bed* provides a peek into the female psyche. I've addressed the most common questions and complaints from men and included feedback from lots of women. Positive responses and techniques used by men to please women are also included in their own words. While I hate stereotyping either sex, I'll acknowledge the more common belief systems, expectations, needs, and ways of thinking in order to help you understand the dynamics between men and women. I'll tell you as honestly as I can how we tick, think, crave sex, have aversions to sex, and drive ourselves crazy over you. Please be patient with us. We all have a long way to go, but it's possible to reach a comfortable compromise.

If you avoid self-help and therapy at any cost (more in Chapter 1), the cost can be your present relationship, or a potential one with a wonderful, supportive, loving partner. A stereotypical guy loves having tools to make and fix things. Think of this book as providing tools in the form of knowledge, understanding, and practical tips for getting along better with women. I know we can be difficult, but there are reasons and possible compromises.

Open up a little and you may learn something. You see, when you take the time to please a woman, she'll probably please *you* a lot more. We love giving when we don't feel we're being taken for granted. We love catering to someone we care about when he's being considerate. We especially love giving pleasure when we're getting satisfied in bed. One man told me, "If you satisfy a woman first, she'll give you much more in return." It often works like that. Give us satisfying sex and many of us will go out of our way to blow your minds.

When you treat us well, you have the best chance of getting the royal treatment in return.

I'm straightforward in this book. You may blush and I may even shock a few of you, but you'll get honesty. I interviewed men and women to get a wide perspective on where the confusion lies, on both sides of the fence (and the bed), and offer suggested solutions. Lots of goodies, tricks, and alternate ways of dealing with your partner have been included. If the old ways aren't working, why not try something new? A self-help book won't kill you, although it might help kill some problems in your relationship and add some spice to your life. Win us over with an understanding of our needs, instead of ignoring or responding to us with scorn or denial.

Read this book and learn new approaches to old problems. Try it. You'll like having her nag less and smile more. Try it. You may enjoy going out with friends when she's not on your case all the time. Try it. You may feel relieved knowing your woman isn't an irrational nut case when you see where her insecurity comes from. Try it. I know you'll love the possibility of having more sex and enjoying it more because you finally know what she wants. Try it. A little more relaxation in a relationship won't hurt you! You may spend less energy trying to please her because what you do will be effective the first time!

How to Please a Woman In & Out of Bed, 2nd Edition is dedicated to all the men who have taken my classes, and those of you concerned enough to read this book. It takes courage for men to break away from old patterns and open themselves up to working on their personal growth. I applaud all of you!

WHY UPGRADE YOUR SOFTWARE?
THE BENEFITS OF CHANGE AND UNDERSTANDING

You're seeing a woman you really like. She seems different from other women you've been involved with. You're determined to get it right this time! You make an effort to call regularly, take her to nice places, and do things to show you care. You go out of your way to help her in any way you can. But just as your pride in yourself is peaking, she accuses you of not communicating, being controlling, and acting as though you don't care. You ask yourself, How could this be? What's wrong with me? What do women want? Do I have to do everything her way if I want to be with her? Can I ever get it right? ～

Do you enjoy, or want to enjoy women? If you do, let's get along better! It's not hard with the right tools and an understanding of where our habits come from. If you can't relate to what we do, it pushes your buttons big time. Hey, you push our buttons too! I'll help you understand our differences and idiosyncrasies. I sincerely believe that when you know where they come from, your response can be less rigid.

Many of you react to problems with women by ignoring them. That often ticks us off more. But you weren't born with the software to deal with us complicated creatures. Do you prefer NOT to do things our way? Well, you don't have to! This book teaches you to create your *own* way that works. Some of the stuff I talk about won't be new to you, but bear with me. I'll try to put a new spin on some played-out topics. Let the potential for much better and more frequent sex motivate you to get through some of the tougher topics. PAY ATTENTION NOW—SMILE LATER!

This chapter explains why you may need to be more equipped to get along better with women. There are many reasons why opening yourself up to the suggestions in this book will benefit you. Here's a few:

1. *You'll feel in control of yourself with women:* We're learning skills for getting what we want faster than you can ignore us. Since we want you, it puts you at a disadvantage if you have no tools for getting your own needs met with us. Controlling yourself, instead of trying to control her, gets you more of what you want. I want you to be as happy as possible!

2. *You'll feel in control of your emotional reactions:* We have a support system for dealing with emotional issues and you don't. Getting tools for handling us in ways that make you healthier and more productive is more satisfying than defending yourself against the repercussions of acting out your fears, anger, or hurt feelings. It's not so hard once you find your own way with my techniques!

3. *You'll have more effective responses to the questions, needs, and accusations women may throw at you:* We ask for a lot. There are little things that can appease our demands and take the pressure off you. I'll give you many simple ways to make us happy so you can enjoy life more fully with a satisfied, secure woman!

4. *You'll be able to do more of the solo activities women complain about:* We may want more time with you than you want with us. Doing things with your friends or on your own can be like going to war. Your life can be more fun when you understand why we need so much from you and learn to help us compromise—without your need for space becoming a major issue.

5. *Hotter and more frequent sex is a likely result of pleasing your woman out of bed:* We're often not as into sex as you are. When you make us happy by meeting some of our pressing needs, which often requires minimal effort, we may be more amenable to making love. I want you to have a great sex life!

6. *Hotter and more frequent sex is a likely result of pleasing your woman in bed:* A woman's body is complicated. By learning its dynamics, you can increase your partner's pleasure in bed by 1000 percent. I'll give you loads of sizzling tools for achieving this. I want you to have more fulfilling sex! I want you to smile more!

Getting Along with Women on Your Own Terms

We do things that appear silly to you. We need things that seem irrational. We can't make up our minds. We pout, we nag, we complain. Okay, some of us are guilty as charged. But don't forget all the good stuff we bring you. It's a balance. Knowing where what you don't like about us comes from helps you handle it. I encourage you *not* to change because we demand it. Improve for YOU! When you take control of *you* and *your* needs, it often improves other arenas of your life as well. You can't positively change anyone but you. (I emphasize this to women, too.) You might bully her for a while or coerce her by playing on her need for a man. But in the long run, that won't nurture love and happiness. I'll provide tools for making your partner happier that are within your comfort zone and won't sell your own needs short. I believe the keys to pleasing women are understanding and compassion.

UNDERSTANDING

Getting along better with us begins with understanding. Insight into where her actions, reactions, and needs come from helps you see they're not necessarily irrational, unfair, or impossible to placate. A good way to know another person is to put yourself in her shoes. I'll ask you regularly to try looking at things from our side, so you'll *know* us better. Then it's easier to accept our needs and actions.

Understanding is a catalyst of change in relationships. You're more pragmatic and have to know "why?" before taking it seriously. I intend to spell out why women are the way we are so you can truly know us vis-à-vis your understanding. Then you'll stop thinking we're nuts and see that we have legitimate, logical reasons for our insecurities, agendas, and fears. This understanding can move you to compassion.

COMPASSION

Your most important tool is here, guys. The key to getting along better with us is compassion. Compassion is using your understanding to develop more patience, tolerance, and empathy for our needs instead of just shrugging them off as "woman things." If you can develop or increase your ability to have compassion for your partner, everything else can fall into place. It's *the* critical skill needed for a successful relationship. Compassion is the lubrication for other tools. The engine of a car freezes up and can't function without oil. Your emotions and responses respond the same way without compassion.

What's compassion? My interpretation of compassion in a relationship is separating actions and situations from caring about your partner's well-being or happiness. It's thinking "I may not agree with her needs but since they're important to her and I love her, I'll make an effort to compromise." When you understand where her needs and actions come from, your capacity for compassion increases. Gordon was excited at a group after learning this:

> *I've always joined my friends making fun of women. We joke that they're irrational with emotions. We imitate them fishing for compliments and speak of them as inferior. You know—the macho thing. I never understood why women are different and that things they do that annoy us were shoved on them. I never thought about why they have hang-ups. Frankly, before this group I never cared. I felt superior to my wife and liked it. Now I understand her more. You're right, I love her and want to make her happy. I used to balk at giving compliments. Now I understand her need for them, so I try. I like being able to please her in ways that are more comfortable for me. I used to think compassion was a woman's word. Now thinking about how much I care for her motivates me to make her happy. Understanding why she asks for certain things sparked my compassion. I know now she's not unreasonable—she's just following her program. I can't tell my friends I have a toolbox full of techniques for getting along better with my wife, but I like knowing it. You emphasized that a lot of what bothers women that we do isn't good for us*

either. I agree. Being conscious of my anger helped me stop taking it out on my wife. I've found better ways to handle it and we talk more. I can't believe how happy we are since I began to take her needs more seriously.

Are you starting to get it? You can become a healthier person for **you**, and your partner, without working too hard or changing who you are. I'll give you the understanding—why we do things that make you crazy; why we ask for what makes no sense to you; why we nag and let emotions control our decisions; why we need so much reinforcement; why we often can't seem to help any of it. You can set your own actions and limitations. Jason called after a seminar:

I thought you were nuts when you introduced Guybercize. My brother dragged me to your workshop and I was skeptical at best. The whole process seemed silly. Why can't men just be men? Well I get it now! I can't believe how differently I'm seeing my girlfriend. I used to just pay her lip service when she'd go on. Now I listen and I'm getting to know her in ways I never thought possible. We talk more. She's respecting my feelings too and not asking for as much as she used to. It's cool having something just for guys. I'd never try a conventional class or book. That's for women. They've been getting too much support for their empowerment while we've had none. Now I feel empowered. Learning how to fix problems with my girl and not feel like I've sold out is empowering!

Compassion enables you to be more sensitive to our needs and feelings. Understanding us with compassion allows you choices— you know how your actions or lack of response makes us feel. Jenna said, "I want a man who knows how to retain his manhood and strength, while still being a compassionate human being." Sensitivity to our feelings makes you a stronger, not weaker man. Compromise isn't changing who you are. You'll never find a "perfect" woman, just as you're not perfect. Caring involves accepting your partner's less appealing qualities and finding ways to deal with them, for both sexes. If they annoy you so much that you can't muster compassion, you shouldn't be with her.

Connection Tip

Look into her eyes and just smile. If she asks why, just say it's because you're happy.

Finding Your Comfort Zone

Why do many of you have difficulty asking for help? We yakity yak regularly to almost anyone who'll listen, about things you wouldn't say to your best friend. Okay, we go overboard sharing problems. Don't emulate us. But until you find your own way to handle problems, they'll perpetually simmer between you and your partner, keeping you from being as happy as possible. You've complained that there are many organizations to support and empower women and none for you. But you act as though you don't need any! Open yourself up and you'll feel more powerful in dealing with us. Let me help you find your way!

STUBBORN INDEPENDENCE

Some of you have always kept what you determined to be your inadequacies to yourself. Growing up, you got subtle—or not so subtle—messages to fix your own problems. You tell me you feel embarrassed, inadequate, and/or ashamed to get help. Many of you would rather lose a woman than ask for advice. Kate told me:

> Shane would rather die than admit he can't handle something. His brother, who was his business partner, died recently. Shane's been clammed up since. I know he's grieving a lot but he won't speak of it. He's been snapping at everyone and going through his own personal hell. He pushes me away when I console him. Shane's dad would help him with the business for a while but he says he can handle it himself. He can't. His foreman told me Shane isn't familiar enough with certain procedures but he's too stubborn to ask for help. So the business is suffering and Shane is suffering, because he can't accept help. He's trying to prove his manhood when he should be grieving the loss of a brother!

Some of you warned me that the hardest part about this book might be getting you to acknowledge that you may have a problem, you're not perfect, SHE may not be fully responsible for tension between you, and your way may not be 100 percent right. Please guys, hear me out! Lighten up a bit. We'll still love you if you remove the Krazy Glue from your blinders and peek at your interaction with us. Actually, we'll probably give you more love, sex, and cooperation if you do.

You're known for being in denial about having problems. I'm being up-front here—be a man and listen! This is just between you and me: Without problems you wouldn't be human. Women sometimes see a computer as more human than you. You know that's ridiculous, but many of you won't admit to being at least partly responsible for problems in your relationship, making it hard to improve things. If you acknowledge problems, you might feel obligated to solve them. Until now you haven't had relationship tools so it was easier to deny they existed. Glenda relayed her experience when she finally got her husband, Jim, to go for marriage counseling:

> Jim reluctantly agreed to go. I was already in therapy but Jim needed to be involved to save our marriage. Jim mainly complained about me. After the first session, Ms. M., our counselor, said, "You should go for individual therapy." Jim smugly announced he knew that I needed help and I was already in therapy. I almost fell off my chair laughing when Ms. M. told him, "I wasn't speaking to her. I was speaking to you." Jim was shocked and defended how much he puts into the relationship and insisted I was the one at fault. Ms. M. explained that a relationship is two people and that I was already working on my issues. She encouraged him to at least acknowledge he had some too. So far he hasn't.

Problems in relationships aren't about who's to blame. Kids point fingers at each other to avoid punishment. But we're not kids. Think of problems as situations instead of making them personal. If she's nagging a lot, the problem isn't her. It's what her nagging and your response to it are doing to your relationship. If you need space and she can't handle it, the problem isn't you. It's what your cooling down and her response to it are doing to your relationship. Think in terms of actions instead of *her* or *me*.

A relationship is two people and their "stuff" interacting. If one party is doing something that the other can't handle, the problem is on both sides. Working together to find more comfortable ways of dealing with each other's "stuff" creates more harmony than pointing fingers. Remember, when there's a problem between two people, both are involved. That means you're involved too! Women aren't to blame for all problems. You need outlets for your emotions and right now don't have many healthy, *manly* ones. Maybe that's why absurd numbers of men physically abuse their families. It may seem more manly to beat a woman than to sit down and discuss problems.

EMOTIONAL BACKLOG

Since we function more emotionally than many of you (more in Chapter 5), women have outlets for letting things out and moving on. Most of us have a support system of friends to work through problems. Dealing with problems is hard if you have no tools, and many of you have empty relationship toolboxes. Bob shared in a class:

> I've been with Bonnie for two years. She wants me to talk about our relationship but I avoid it. Things are wrong but I don't know what to do. Talking makes me angry. She knows exactly what's screwing up and what to do about it. I don't see things like her so I tune out. My dad said that's how women are—they like to analyze and work on improving what can be left alone. I don't know. She wants to go for couples therapy but no way! I can't even talk to Bonnie, so how can I talk about my failures to a stranger? I feel like a failure—I don't know how to help our relationship. I don't want to lose Bonnie. Things probably would work in a better way if I could think of solutions like she does. I don't like listening to her when I feel lost. So she keeps talking and I keep ignoring her.

Does this sound familiar? You can feel like a failure if you have no solution. That's unfair to you! You weren't given tools to fix relationships! You've been told self-help books and classes aren't for men. "Men should find a solution on their own." That's crap and you know it! No one can know everything. Although the *solve it myself* attitude is changing, I bet most of you choose to blindly "handle" women dilemmas yourself, with little satisfaction. Since traditionally you've avoided self-help like the plague, a majority of you still turns your back on it.

THE RELIEF OF SHARING

The tone of my workshops for men is different. Women are shocked to hear that there's more bonding and camaraderie. Guys love hearing others share the same fears and frustrations they have. Once they get comfortable, the guys are eager to express themselves and be enlightened. Some of them have been in therapy. Most haven't. For many of them, my forum is their first opportunity to attempt some personal growth. Jackie admitted in a class:

> My dad discouraged complaining about what I couldn't do, saying, "Find a way to work it out." He'd tell my mom to ignore my asking for advice with school problems. As I got older there was pressure to do well on my own. I resented my dad but never had the balls to challenge him. I still have an aversion to asking for help. My wife gets mad if I clam up about problems. She tried getting me to couples counseling but how could I? I know my dad was wrong but I can't talk about anything serious. I wish I could. I came to this class out of desperation, for a different way to handle problems. It's a relief to see so many of you have trouble with problems and also want to change. I thought something was wrong with me. It's hard to unlearn what was forced on me for thirty years.

Do you think you're the only one wanting to express your feelings but can't? Lighten up on yourself. A majority of men share your inability to step outside walls built in childhood. They also feel funny about not having a solution for pleasing us. Sure, you can yes us to death to get us off your backs or momentarily appease us, but becoming more enlightened can be a relief.

MEN AND WOMEN AND PERSONAL GROWTH

My male students all want to know what women want and how to please them. They feel inadequate in bed and want to learn how to deal with women on all levels. Women want tools for dealing with friends, family, and colleagues. You just want to talk about us. You ask a zillion questions about pleasing us. We discuss; we suggest; we encourage; we support. You don't understand why we can't accept your difficulty in opening up. But we don't get it. Claudia asked me:

> Why do men have so much trouble talking to us? I can't get any boyfriend to speak openly about problems. My girlfriends and I always discuss this. We talk out problems and find solutions. Men seem to avoid everything, which muddles up the relationship. It's so easy to say what's on your mind. Why can't men do it? And why do they have so much trouble listening objectively? When I try to discuss something with my current guy, he shuts down, gets defensive, and I can't get through. What's wrong with men?

Nothing is wrong with you. We just express ourselves more easily. That doesn't make one sex right or wrong. But we can make you feel wrong. We get frustrated when you won't talk out problems. We push you to open up. We nag. We complain. We withhold sex. When you can't deal with our frustration, you may do something that annoys us more. It's much more fun to break the cycle.

Why Do I Need Help with Women?

We think, react, communicate, and have needs that can seem completely contrary on the surface. It can work if we respect each other. Staying in the same place, and denying problems won't make relations between the sexes better. A change of direction might. Your road map is on the following pages.

Male Bonding versus Female Bonding

Women like to bond over the misery of breaking up, gaining weight, problems on the job, serious shopping as well as other issues in their lives. You bond over a six-pack, a ball game, music, a discussion about politics. We love each other, hate each other, and are jealous of each other. Many of you probably don't get nearly that deep with each other. You're probably content to just hang and have fun. We can't relate to how many of you find it hard to connect on an emotional level, since we do it so naturally.

Talking one-on-one with a friend can be more comfortable. Male bonding can take on a macho attitude when you hang in a group. Most of you aren't comfortable being the first to admit you have trouble with women. In class, when one man acknowledges having problems with us, the floodgates open—man after man wants a turn talking about his feelings.

Solving Problems

A major difference between men and women is how we handle problems. As you suppress or deny them, we go to the other extreme and overanalyze. I believe a major reason for stress between the sexes is that you're *undertherapied* (therapy deprivation) and we're *overtherapied* (therapy overkill). This creates a very unbalanced situation—we're armed to the teeth and all you can do is duck.

Think about it. Most women have always had a form of therapy. Little girls talk out problems with someone older. Our circle of advisors grows as we develop friendships. We work through problems with support from the get-go. Boys are encouraged to keep problems in. You suppress them, cope, and stoically go on rather than find someone to talk to. Little boys with suppressed emotions can grow into men who keep everything in. But feelings that you push aside can eventually come back to haunt you, creating a clash between you and your partner. Dan agreed in a coed support group:

Several women I trusted let me down before so I'm careful now. Women say I'm cold. I'm just trying to protect myself but I don't tell them. So we fight and it ends. Sometimes I think I provoke fights to avoid future problems. I actually bolted on someone I liked a lot—I didn't want to get hurt. She kept calling and I dodged. I felt bad. I wanted to be with her but I'm not ready to put myself on the line. Sometimes I think I'm losing it—splitting from someone I enjoy being with. Jen kept trying to get me to tell her why I seemed scared but I refused to talk. I've done that already and ended up hurt. Now

I want to be in control and the only way is to stay on top of my feelings. I couldn't with Jen, so I left.

Dan handled his fear of getting hurt by avoiding intimacy. Guys, you can fix cars, do well at work, and find practical solutions for daily problems. But when dealing with us, there's no contest on who's better equipped to cope on an emotional front. We're learning, growing, and trying on new hats. Thanks to classes, books, friends, and therapy, we can handle almost anything—except you! We go overboard trying to analyze, change, and understand you while many of you go overboard avoiding a confrontation.

As we struggle to get in touch with our inner child so that we can grow up, many of you are trying to hold on to your inner child so you don't have to. Over 75 percent of the women I interviewed said they'd been in therapy. About 25 percent of you had gotten outside help with problems. A large percentage of your therapy was couples counseling at your partner's insistence. Do you see why the level of coping with relationship issues between the sexes can be unbalanced?

Better interaction between us starts with respecting each other's right to be different. You don't have to do all the bending. I encourage women to accept you as you are too. Get your partner to read *All Men Are Jerks Until Proven Otherwise* to get her tools. It's easier to get along if you bring your problems out in the open. Jared called a week after taking a class to share his experience with his partner:

I heard what you said in class but couldn't imagine dealing with Lori differently. The more I thought about your words, the more I wanted to make our relationship work. We had problems—she'd get angry when I ignored her complaints about what I wasn't doing. They seemed endless before your class. Now I see I embellished them as a way of doing nothing about what she didn't like. When I paid attention, I understood Lori didn't complain all the time as I'd convinced myself. But when she told me something, it felt like an ongoing tirade because I had no response. Now I'm trying to actually listen instead of just letting her comments roll off of me. You gave me ways to handle what she's been asking for and I'm making an attempt for the first time in my life. It feels good to not run from problems. I want my relationship to work and now feel more capable of contributing to that happening. I felt scared trying but I'm doing it!

I'll be gentle with you guys! The relief of handling problems instead of handling the repercussions of not dealing with them will make you a lot happier. It should certainly make us happier, which translates into more peace and satisfying rewards for you. Practicing new skills doesn't have to be unpleasant. Allen took my class and asked for a private session with me and his girlfriend, Sue. He'd never been in therapy but wanted to move forward after class. Sue was thrilled. They talked about simple things. They worked on more complex issues. All I did was offer them a comfortable environment to talk in. Allen tried his newly acquired communication skills and Sue readily responded. She told me afterward:

I was amazed when Allen said he was ready to communicate by listening. He admitted he'd felt inadequate before and couldn't discuss anything I brought up. Now he's ready to try. When he asked if we could start with you present, of course I agreed. I'd do almost anything if Allen is trying to work with me. It was great hearing him open up a little in our session. Now I understand why it's been so hard for him and think we'll be okay. I see what I do that closes him up and he sees how much it means to me when he tries. He seems so happy to be able to cope with me. We were on opposite planets before.

You can learn to solve problems. I believe in you! I know you can adopt new tricks for dealing with old problems with your sometimes demanding, irrational, needy, critical partner. I don't recommend major or uncomfortable changes. But understanding why certain methods and words get more for the same mileage may motivate you to try alternatives to what's not working now. Give it a shot. You'll enjoy getting along better!

2 TECHNICAL GLITCHES IN OUR PROGRAMS: MEN AND WOMEN CAN BE COMPATIBLE

You watch your partner in horror as she does things the opposite of how you would. You clench your teeth as she demands a lot more than you feel you should give. She whines and complains when she doesn't get her way. If you do what you know is best for her she gets bent out of shape. What a big deal she makes of having you around! Why can't she be more independent and enjoy autonomy like you do? Why can't she think like men? She needs to learn how but won't listen. You wonder if it's possible for men and women to get along. ～

Both sexes have differences we enjoy and ones we'd prefer didn't exist. You may not like our hidden agendas but enjoy the spice we bring to your life. You may not like our nagging but the differences are applauded when you're horny. Let's face it—you may not always like being with us but you don't want to live without us! Since you can't keep us in bed all the time and we don't live on Fantasy Island, men and women need to learn to balance each other's annoying qualities against the delicious ones. We were programmed from birth on with what we should expect from each other. It's hard to let go of our upbringing. But we can.

Accepting the Differences
It helps to understand the different programs we're brought up with. You're more goal oriented and see your worth in terms of accomplishments.

We learned to please and see our worth in terms of who likes us, most importantly you. You've heard this before. Try to really understand the dynamics this time.

You define yourself by more concrete/fewer personal factors: your income (job), ability to fix something (power), confidence in facing fears, and general achievements. We define ourselves by more personal factors: having a man, knowing people like us, and feeling pretty and thin enough. It's sad that even women with successful careers say that they feel incomplete without a man. We haven't learned as you did to be enthused with accomplishments. Only you make many of us fulfilled. You're the prize, guys, like it or not!

RAISED TO ATTRACT MEN

I find your direction a lot healthier, but we use what we're taught. While you were encouraged to think of careers, we worked on looking good to attract you. Many women got no encouragement to develop a satisfying career. The attitude is changing, but not as much as you'd think. It's hard to stop making you our most important need. Bette explained to a coed group:

> I wanted to be a doctor but was told to go to nursing school. My career was never important. My brother got that support. When we'd visit family, Brian could wear a jacket over jeans. I had to wear a dress and my aunts would notice if I'd gained a pound. Everyone cared how Brian was doing in school and what his goals were. Everyone cared if I had a boyfriend. No one took my desire to be a doctor seriously. Now I'm a nurse and everyone wants to know if I have a potential husband. I'd love to get married since I find nursing unsatisfying. I wish I'd bucked everyone and gone to med school. I'm stuck with no satisfaction. The only approval I can get is for a husband. And Brian is still screwing around from woman to woman— no one cares. Getting married seems all I can do now.

Put yourself in our shoes. This is nothing new but maybe you've never quite understood the pressure on us. Nobody cared if I aspired to serious career goals but someone always watched me eat and warned me about gaining weight or I wouldn't get a boyfriend.

We're pushed to attract you—if we don't, something is wrong with us. Family, friends, and the media say if we don't work hard on our appearance, you won't want us. Then we're nothing. Who we attract is our equivalent of your need to be successful. No matter how happy and successful we are, some people give women without a man pity. Yes, pity. Even happily single women say they have to endure consoling looks and comments from stupid people who can't imagine a woman being happy if she's not in a relationship. It happens to me. Many people can't accept that I'm happy on my own. When I left my last boyfriend, women gave me sympathy instead of patting me on the back for making a healthy choice. I'm finally strong enough to handle this attitude. Most women aren't. Are you getting it? A career is much more satisfying than getting a man, just so we don't look like a loser.

I always wanted a career, but it was drummed into my head that teaching was the **only** acceptable career for a woman. I grew up responding to questions about what I wanted to be with "anything but a teacher!" My school advisor insisted teaching was my best option, despite my argument to study business because of my high math scores. She said I didn't need a career—I'd get a husband to take care of me. I was pushed against my will into Liberal Arts, and ended up a teacher! Then having a man became more important to me (my only option for success). I settled for marriage. Have you ever felt comatose from your career? That's what my "success" did for me.

If we don't get satisfaction from a career, attracting you may be our top achievement. Girls aren't given the choices, confidence, and inspiration boys get automatically. An average man feels validated when he achieves a goal. The ultimate form of validation for an average woman is to be in a successful relationship. And you wonder why we make you so important?

THOSE DARN STEREOTYPES

Girls and boys grow up with different programs, reinforced by parents, friends, teachers, and the media. Each sex develops different attitudes. Trying to change them isn't easy. Georgia said:

I wanted to raise Connie without stereotypes. As a youngster she wore blue overalls and didn't have much hair so people assumed she was a boy. I said nothing. At the playground Connie joined the boys and played rough, which was fine with me. Most girls played quieter. People changed when they knew she was a girl. I got flack for not worrying about her appearance. She was a baby! I wanted to give her choices. Connie loved sports and played with boys at school. I was criticized for that too—I should teach her to stay clean and play nicer! It took years for her to earn respect from boys she played ball with. She's more independent than most girls but teachers don't take her as seriously as boys. I know I did right—Connie has more dreams than all my friends' daughters put together. That's worthwhile!

Years ago on TV, I saw a bald baby brought to two groups of people to play. For the first group, the baby had a girl's name, wore pink, and had a bow around its bald head. The men and women in this first group were gentle. They cooed, calling her *sweet, pretty, a little doll,* in high-pitched voices. The same baby was then dressed in denim and given a boy's name for the second group. They played more roughly, throwing him higher in the air and exerting a lot more energy. They spoke louder, referring to him as a *hearty little guy, a tiger.* This was the same baby!

I remember observing Riva with her young boys when we sat together at a community swimming pool. They ran on concrete, sometimes teetering at the edge of the pool. She explained boys should be allowed to take more chances and added that her sister had it easier with girls. They could be made to sit still. Riva justified, "Boys handle getting hurt better than girls. My mom said I have to give them the freedom to learn for themselves so they don't grow up afraid, because they're boys. Girls, on the other hand, should be kept out of trouble and protected more."

What messages do kids get from these stereotypes? That we trust boys to take care of themselves more than we trust girls. I doubt you can imagine how insecure this attitude makes us. We're regularly reminded that we can't take care of ourselves—we're warned to be careful, not given responsibility, and discouraged from taking risks.

I was fortunate that my dad didn't bring me up this way. I always had a stronger sense of self and less need for guys. I was the only one not obsessed about having a Saturday night date from my early teens on. I was seen as weird when I'd choose to stay home and read a book instead of dating a guy who didn't interest me. My friends dated any old schlep, just to have one.

I hear little boys told "Be a man." Who defined your role? It's like when people say "They say" and no one knows who "they" are. What's a man? Someone cold? Unfeeling? Capable of finding solutions to all problems? Insensitive to women? I've never seen these definitions. Widely held stereotypes often attribute these qualities to men, but are they what defines you? Do you really believe you'll be less of a man if you express your feelings, show sensitivity, or ask for help? Stretch your possibilities and define yourself. A real man chooses his own way based on what feels right, not by what tradition mandates.

 Connection Tip

Give her a deep, loving kiss just before you leave for work. Then look her in the eyes, smile, and leave. You'll be on her mind all day.

ACCEPTANCE

Men and women need to accept each other's right to be who we are. It's our choice to deal with, or not to deal with, each person in our lives. It's not our choice to change them (I emphasize this to women too!). Aren't both sexes entitled to their needs and nuances? There's a difference between things that are unacceptable and those you just don't like. George related to this in a class:

> I liked Tess from the beginning but she got on my nerves. She loved hugging, which I'm not comfortable with, and sometimes she talks too critically about people. Eventually everything she did made me bristle. I'd get on her a lot. She was ready to leave me when my sister noticed and spoke up. Ruth asked what bothered me the most about Tess. Easy—she picked apart my friends. Ruth made me realize my anger about that blew other things out of proportion. I told Tess that what she said about my friends was intolerable and apologized

*for putting down her other habits. Okay, I'm not wild about affec-
tion but that's Tess and I can compromise on more trivial matters.
Ruth taught me to take each case separately and be objective about
whether I have a right to expect her to stop. I'm falling in love with
Tess and getting used to her, as long as she leaves my friends alone.*

Many of you said you don't like being "the stronger sex"; you hate
having to achieve; you'd like to be more comfortable sharing fears
with friends. We didn't choose to be emotional and needy; many of
us would love to enjoy having an autonomous life. It will take time
for both sexes to unlearn what we've been taught. We can get used to
each other and learn to accept that there will be both irritating and
delicious things about us all. Of course if she annoys the heck out of
you, she may not be right for you. But don't look for perfection either.
Too many potentially good relationships get destroyed because one
party refuses to accept the other's ways.

Knowing Better Than Us

Many of you think you can read us well and it shows in your
attitude. Some of you that I spoke to had inflated confidence in your
ability to assess us. I separately interviewed both partners in several
relationships and compared answers. Men were sure they understood
their partner while women said their partners needed help. Andrew
was confused in a class:

*Schuyler gets angry when I finish her sentences but she's so predict-
able. She says I don't know her as well as I think, but I do! I know
what makes her happy and do what's best for her. Schuyler doesn't
appreciate it. She fights me to make decisions for herself when I
know what's best. Women are alike. When my friends and I hang
at the bar, we get a kick out of seeing how similar our girlfriends are.
We have some good laughs over it.*

You may humor us instead of listening. That's disrespectful. You
can go too far with your program to take care of us. We look to you
for security, but want respect for our needs, thoughts, and feelings.
Don't treat us as little girls and tell us what we think. Beth said: "I

had a boyfriend who second-guessed me. He was always wrong, but no matter how often I proved it, he'd finish my next thought. He's lucky his voice isn't high pitched now if you know what I mean!" Male bonding can include making fun of us. You joke about our needs and feelings. That makes you take them even less seriously, which isn't fair.

Satisfying Needs

We don't have more needs than you. In fact, men and women have many needs in common, but we deal with them differently. We all relish getting comfort and support from someone we care about. You may ignore your needs more to avoid seeming unmanly, but both sexes have lots of needs.

Needing Love

Our most common need is for love. Come on, guys, admit it. You need love too. We may show that need more and demand it more, but all human beings want it. Love is nice, good, fun, and essential to our existence. Don't deny that you appreciate love as much as we do. Budd discovered how important love was to him when his girlfriend went away on business:

> Alanna places a high value on love. She romanticizes everything and has loving interaction with everyone close to her. I used to tease her about it and she'd say she felt sorry for me not appreciating how great love was. When her boss asked her to move to Dallas for six months, I wasn't happy but couldn't stand in her way. She didn't want to leave and be without my love but I encouraged her to go. She said I was cold and I laughed, so she went. Well she had the last laugh. I felt awful without her. I wanted to beg her to come home but couldn't. I was more lovesick than she, flying to see her a few times a month. Alanna was shocked. So was I. We make fun of how women do so much for love but Alanna said we're bigger babies about needing love and I'm thinking she's right.

Martin added:

After my last relationship ended, I missed loving a woman. I wanted it so badly I was embarrassed. My friends would have thought I was lame if they knew how much I missed love. I spoke to a female friend who said she liked hearing a guy admit what we all must feel. She said women have more comfortable sources of love than we do. They hug and kiss friends, family—even strangers. We don't, so we don't express love as much. Maybe we need it more. I missed like crazy my ex's loving nature for comfort, and of course sex.

We let our needs hang out while you do your best to keep us from knowing you have them too. Some of you see admitting a need for love as a weakness. But it can be a strength when you find a comfortable way to express it. Love does rule, so when it happens, why not relax and enjoy it?

Since our world often revolves around you, our needs do too. While you fought off hugs and kisses as kids, we relished being coddled, pampered, and lavished with affection. Many of you still fight hugs and kisses—we still relish being coddled, pampered, and lavished with affection. Then we get hurt and frustrated if you seem to not care.

No matter how strong, successful, or independent we are, love is essential for our well-being. But we don't always keep this need in perspective. Women in movies get ridiculous amounts of romance/attention/affection/adoration. We want it too! In romance novels, lovers use most of their energy giving love. The concepts we learn in fiction are incredibly appealing. But real life isn't fiction. Many of us fantasize Prince Charming sweeping us off our feet and loving us intently. Watching our parents, friends, and other real-life partners isn't as exciting. So we dream about fiction while reality frustrates us. Janice wrote me:

I've been waiting for my prince my whole life. I've always lost myself in romance novels. No one lived up to my fantasy men. I honestly couldn't separate fact from fiction and thought I was just meeting bad ones. After reading All Men Are Jerks Until Proven Otherwise *I see my expectations have been fictitious. I forced myself to stop the novels and wrote a list of what was most important in a man. I'm seeing a guy now who isn't my prince but gives me a lot of what I need. Now that I'm back to reality, I can appreciate a guy who isn't a perfect romantic. I still wish there were men who could be like the ones in books and movies but I'm learning not to need so much and can enjoy real life more.*

Nurture-Mania

Do you enjoy loving attention and the little things we do to show we care? Of course you do. We love nurturing you—you love being nurtured. Accept it. Many of you admit you thoroughly enjoy it when we act like a lady-in-waiting and treat you like a prince. So why do you bristle when we'd like those goodies too?

It's funny how things you love getting from us are often those you gripe about when we want them from you. When we lavish you with loving gestures it feels good. Think about it. Your ego is boosted when we compliment you or let you know we care. You take pleasure in being coddled, lovingly handled, and catered to. So why are we seen as pains in the butt if we want some?

 Connection Tip

After work, massage her shoulders, rub your fingers in circles on her temples and jawbone to melt tension away.

Turning Demands into Smiles

You complain that women are demanding creatures, and we can be at times. You complain we need more than you could ever satisfy. Wrong! We may ask for the sun, the moon, and the stars, but we'd settle for a lot less. Learning to appease some of our more pressing needs results in a happier partner. The little things I speak of in the following pages can be the keys to pleasing us. You can put a minimum amount of effort into keeping us happy enough to go to the ends of the earth, not to mention the bed, for you! Throughout this book I'll refer to little things that can make us feel special. Never forget that most women who feel happy and satisfied will want to reciprocate since we're giving by nature. Make us all happy by stimulating us to give!

WHAT'S THE BIG DEAL?

Our need for you to acknowledge our existence gets blown out of proportion. While we can make too big a deal with our cry for attention, satisfying us can be the simplest thing you ever do. The rewards can be so great that you'll wish you'd learned to please us sooner!

What you see as a need for attention is often a need to feel a connection, a link to you. We crave intimacy and closeness but don't express it clearly. You interpret it as being needy for attention. It's not. Connections to those we care about are important to us—one of the most important needs you can satisfy. Easily!

We've had connections with friends since childhood, and especially need to feel connected to you. They let us know we're on your radar screen, especially when you're wrapped up in work or needing space. Studies show that couples with the best relationships are those who maintain connections. It shows us you care when you do things to connect, even if it's not what *you* need. Couples can stay connected without a major effort.

LITTLE THINGS THAT CREATE A CONNECTION

Touch

Any form of touching can strengthen our connection *and* keep you healthier for the same price. Studies show that regular tactile contact is imperative for our well-being—both men and women. This includes hugging, squeezing, caressing, massaging—any touching. Extended periods of touch are most beneficial but any touch contact can maintain the all-important connection we need. Robert said:

Mandi and I work at home. We each have our own area in the same room and respect each other's need for space when working. But whenever she gets up, she walks by and makes contact. Sometimes it's a quick kiss—a pinch—a brush on my body lightly with her hand as she walks by. I always smile at what she does and recently told her that. She said that was her way of keeping connected to me. I liked that. She asked me to remember how nice it feels when I get up. Now I do it to Mandi too. It does make me feel closer to her.

A slight touch during a busy day keeps connections solid. We may allow you more space if we feel connected. When a former boyfriend and I read the Sunday paper in bed, he'd lie in the opposite direction, at my feet. I did everything I could to connect with him, but he ignored me. Normally, he was all over me, so I felt especially disconnected Sunday mornings. I explained my need—he said he liked reading in peace and accused me of being high maintenance because I needed this attention. Most of the time he suffocated me yet when I expressed my need for a connection I was unfairly labeled. I'd have accepted him rubbing my toe or an occasional grunt in my direction, just to acknowledge my presence. Honestly, a simple toe touch would have appeased me. Little things can get big results!

 Connection Tip

Share a package of your favorite candies or sweets that you both like. Feed each other.

Words

Some sweet words can keep connections solid—a quick phone call at work—a loving thought whispered in public—saying "I'll miss you" when you go on a business trip—a word of encouragement—compliments—these can all go far. Benny said, "It's a relief to see my wife doesn't need too much from me to feel close. I've made an effort to say nice things at least once a day. She says it means a lot to her. You were right, it only takes a little!"

Notes

A note or card is a great way to strengthen a connection. It doesn't have to be a love note, though "I love you" will be well received. Try a smiley face with your initial slipped into her book—a loving thought on a Post-It on the mirror—a provocative suggestion for activities later in her handbag. The Internet makes it easy for those of you online. A short e-mail to say you're thinking of her takes little time and connects us. Cheryl said, "What endeared Barry to me were his little messages. When we first met it was e-mails saying

'Hope you're having a great day.' I never know where I'll find a sweet note. It's intensified our bond and makes me secure. I've saved them all. They're worth more than diamonds!" (and cheaper!)

Gestures

Connections are created by many kinds of gestures—eyes meeting in a group—helping us with a problem—accompanying us to an event that's important to us—doing something as soon as we ask—things that say you care. A boyfriend bought me a water filter when there were warnings about our water—our connection intensified from that loving gesture. Little things you do that show you took the time to please us mean the most. Jane said, "Peter cut out a sentimental comic strip that related to feelings we've shared and left it under my pillow when he knew we wouldn't see each other for a few days. It made me feel closer to him and I always take it out when he's not here. It reminds me he cares."

Rituals

I'd like to introduce you to something that some of you may think of as a "woman thing"—rituals. A ritual in a relationship is something you do regularly—meditating together for five minutes before sleep, washing each other's hair on Saturday, touching base every day by phone at the same time, eating dinner by candlelight on Thursdays, taking walks, renting a movie on Tuesday nights, cooking a meal together each week, exchanging massages on Sunday. Shared rituals keep connections strong in a hectic world. Craig said, "Bonnie puts a little treat in my lunch bag every day. It's always a surprise. It might be cookies, an exotic fruit, a note, a silly windup toy. It doesn't matter what. It reminds me Bonnie cares and she knows I think of her every day at lunch."

Connections give us reassurance and help us feel closer to you. They tell us you care, and that you pay attention to what we like and how we think. Creating a connection doesn't take effort and it can deepen a relationship. When you're wrapped up in activities that don't involve your lady, connections let her know you're still thinking about her, even if you ignore her most of the time. Although some of us love getting gifts of jewelry, flowers, and other material things, little things make many of us happier. The little, thoughtful things you do to show you care are the most meaningful.

You should enjoy giving us some of what we want if you care. We can learn to be happy with what you're capable of giving. I'll point out more of these little things that can make a big difference in later chapters. You want a good relationship? You want a happy lady? Next time she says she needs to feel connected, drop the ball and chain image. Ask what you can do. I can't emphasize enough it's the little things that will give you the most peace. A small bit of attention given freely can have tremendous results!

Working with Our Differences

When we first fall for someone, annoying quirks, expectations, and differences are often tolerated since we're on our best behavior. So she's a bit demanding—look how cute she is. Later they become unacceptable. Understanding them can help you accept us more as we are.

Keeping Your Inner Child to Yourself

We please others. You're known for putting yourself first. We worry more about everyone. Women complain you can get very self-absorbed and forget there are two people in a relationship. It's fine to make you the number one priority of your world. I encourage women to do that. But we can't revolve exclusively around you in a good relationship. You may get away with it at first but not forever. Teddy learned the hard way:

> When my fiancé moved in, she did what I expected. After a few weeks she said while she didn't mind being good to me, it felt like both of us worried about me. I made a joke out of it and Celia stopped doing stuff. I got nasty. Other girlfriends had gone along with me so why not my future wife? She called me a spoiled brat, said I didn't take life seriously, and there was no room for her needs. She gave me back the ring and said she was moving. I woke up. I have been spoiled in the past, but never loved anyone like I love Celia.

I want to make her happy too. Women have said they were happy if they pleased me. I took it as my due as the man. I begged Celia for another chance. She's staying but won't wear the ring till she sees I'm serious. Now I do as much for her as she does for me.

We joke that you still like being little boys—except it's not funny. Your mothers may have catered to you and girlfriends followed suit. Some of you get spoiled and expect us to indulge your whims. I love letting the little girl in me come out to play. It makes life more fun. But the child in us shouldn't play at someone else's expense. Acting like a child makes you take life less seriously. It helps you forget responsibilities for a time. That's fine when you're out with the other boys but it can screw up a relationship if you do it too often.

THOSE DARN SHTICKS

Sometimes we think in opposite directions. Refusing to budge makes it harder to work together. You may see asking for help as not being in control. We feel more in control if we ask. You see it as a weakness—you want results on your own. We feel it's an accomplishment to ask for and get what we need. Not knowing it all doesn't make you less of a man. Getting answers from others makes you more of one since your know-how increases! We know you'd rather drive for hours than get directions. If you have time and gas, enjoy the ride. When I get lost I head for the nearest gas station, to get where I'm going faster. That's more satisfying to me than driving through two extra states to find my way. I'm not criticizing your right or need to do this. Just be aware that getting assistance from others can aid you without compromising your masculinity. Jay called after a class:

I wanted you to know I asked for help several times this weekend. It started as an experiment—homework from your class. Saturday my car was knocking. Normally I'd have spent all day if necessary fixing it myself. But I thought of how much other work I had and remembered what you said about saving time by asking so I called a friend to stop by—he found the problem right away. It was good having time to do what I'd intended. When Lisa and I went to visit her cousin upstate on Sunday I got lost. Normally I'd have struggled with a map for hours while Lisa fumed. She was shocked when I pulled into a gas station and got directions. We got there fast. I realize I've been stubborn about doing things myself. This weekend turned out to be very relaxing. I'll probably ask for help again some time!

 Connection Tip

Whistle at her when she comes out of the shower.

Try it. You may be pleasantly surprised by the result! In the past, your ways were considered better. You may prefer them, which is fine. But our personal, intuitive, and detailed approach has proven effective. There's more than one way to do things. Respecting each other's right to their own approach will make us more compatible. Sherman explained how his problems with his wife became lessons:

When I first lived with Marley I put her down because she did things differently from me. It was a definite macho thing. She'd take time to evaluate decisions while I jumped in. She managed to get support for projects at work using her people skills, which I thought of then as a waste of time. Marley got so fed up with my poking fun at her that she almost moved out. That made me do a reality check. I fell in love with her because of who she is. People like her more than me. She's had more promotions. I paid attention to how she handled people and tried doing some of it. I learned patience and kindness from Marley. It's paid off at my job. Guess an old dog can learn some new tricks—even from a woman!

We can learn from each other and absorb qualities by watching each other with respect. If couples communicate about differences, they can be softened. Watch your partner implement her strong traits and encourage her to do the same. Let her teach you personal skills. Appreciate some of the things you balk at. Learning from each other is a growth process for both sexes. Robert wrote:

I think men in general need to be more in touch with how society forms who and what we are. They also need to learn what real trust and responsibility is. Most of all, they need to treat women the way they would want to be treated.

Taking Control of Your Choices

Men regularly complain that they always meet the same type of woman. That's not an accident. I strongly believe that we get back what we expect. While we may not like the qualities, both men and women are attracted to what's familiar. You have a defense system in place for certain types. For example, if you keep ending up in relationships with needy women, it's because you're used to that and expect to meet them. If you want a different type, get conscious about what you expect women to be.

Jerry wrote to me after the first edition of this book, saying, "My experience is that women generally place a very high value on a man's financial security abilities and also having the means to entertain at an ability that is totally unreasonable." He expects women to want him for security and they do. I know lots of men who are surprised about women wanting that, because they never meet those types. Yet Jerry gives out something that attracts more materialistic women to him. He told me about his financial situation, even to the car he drives, when he described himself. I encouraged him to forget those things when meeting women and stick to who he is as a person. EXPECT to meet someone different! If you recognize the signs in her earlier, be strong and move on. Some people only date security seekers, or alcoholics, or frigid women. Find your pattern and think about why you end up with this type. Consciously prevent it the next time. Don't keep staying with women that remind you of those before. Be aware that not every woman you meet will be right for you, and that's okay.

You only need to meet one person for a relationship. There can be two thousand or two million "Ms. Wrongs." You only need one "Ms. Right." Focus on that. It doesn't matter how many women don't work out. Work on your spirituality and focus on only needing to meet one good woman. If you have faith that when the time is right you'll meet someone special, you can relax and enjoy your life more. When you're ready for a relationship, you'll find her.

3

Decoding Our Mixed Signals:
The Rationale Behind What Seems Irrational

You call the woman you're dating to follow through on plans you'd discussed last week. Now she's not sure. You ask what she wants and she asks what you want. Your patience dwindles as she has no answer. Then she jumps down your throat for pressuring her to do something that was her idea in the first place! You step back and she asks if you're still interested in her—she needs you to act more enthusiastic about making plans. You advise her to think about your conversation and she coldly says she doesn't need you to tell her what to do. When you ask her to lighten up, she hangs up. What do women want? Are they all nuts? You feel like kicking a wall from the exasperation she provokes in you. ❧

Women can say one thing and mean another. "No" can mean "yes." Our signals may seem irrational to your more practical side. We waffle between what we want and what we think we should do. I know we can be exasperating. It takes patience and compassion to handle our mixed signals. Many factors affect our response to simple things. PMS, our friend's influence, horniness, guilt about being horny, going to a wedding, and stress in general contribute to what you deal with.

Soothing Uptight Women

Everyone influences our thoughts and actions. Since our sense of self is often tied to you, your importance is inflated. Our lack of autonomy puts too much pressure on you. We're trying to change, but our upbringing that told us to please others affects many of our decisions, or our inability to make them.

WE'RE RIGHT/ YOU'RE WRONG!

You ask if I believe you're as wrong as women make you feel. We may criticize what seems like your every move. We look for trouble and let you know when we find it. Some of you must feel like a target in a shooting gallery, dodging bullets in the form of words from us. Sound familiar? Brad complained:

> *I give up! My girlfriend always gets on me for something. I don't call enough. I don't make enough time for her. She dislikes my wardrobe. And on and on. I don't know what to do. She makes me feel like I can't do anything right. She's not the first to do it. I hear it from friends too. Women can make us feel like we're defective or something . . . like they do it right and we do it wrong. And they wonder why we don't spend more time with them.*

We give mixed signals as we struggle to find ourselves. We're used to following rules as part of our "good girl" program. Girls grow up making group decisions. Many of us still have the old software. You're more action oriented and solve problems while we worry about possible outcomes. If you act unconcerned, we think you don't care. We want you to worry with us. We dwell on what we're scared about and take it out on you. Many of us—men and women—watched our parents in these roles and followed in their footsteps.

 Connection Tip

Put some heart candies, a heart lollipop, or some candy kisses in her pocket, briefcase, or lunch.

We want help but need to maintain our domain. Have you tried doing a chore and had your partner take over? Does she act like you don't diaper the baby properly, get dishes clean, or do laundry right? Just as fixing things is your domain, domestic matters are ours. We

complain if you don't do enough and butt in when you do—we think
we do it better. Sound familiar? It's hard for some of us to let go of an
area we want to control. Ask us to show you how rather than take it
over. Say you'd like to keep trying until you get it right.

DIFFERENT PERCEPTIONS

We analyze you to death trying to understand you. If you don't
see our point, you may label it dumb and move on. We waste energy
trying to make you understand and get upset if you don't respond.
You're more practical and need to understand before accepting it.
We'd rather you go along with us. Period. You state something con-
cretely. If you don't relate, you can't take our needs seriously and may
label them as "women stuff," treat them as trivial, or just ignore them.
We may not know how to explain what we want in terms that you
understand. Some of you give us messages that you don't want to
know anyway. Manny told a group:

> When Kenya got mad if I watched TV or read during dinner, I'd
> ignore her. She'd make a fuss and I'd tune out. I thought she was
> a typical woman, picking on trivia. She'd say it was important to
> interact at dinner but I never understood. I thought she was try-
> ing to control me and I rebelled. One night we talked about her
> parents' divorce. She said one of the reasons her mom left her dad
> was she couldn't connect with him because he ignored them at what
> she'd been brought up to think of as family times, like dinner. Kenya
> wanted that time with me, thinking our marriage might fall apart
> otherwise. It makes sense now and I save things for after dinner. If
> only women made their needs clear!

You need clear explanations. But many of us don't have the skills
to spell it out and many of you don't have the patience or know-how
to pull it out of us. It's especially hard when things that bother us
wouldn't bother you. Sexuality is a good example. We hate feeling
like a sex object because we've had bad experiences with men who
treated us like we didn't matter beyond sex. Many of you would
love a woman to say she'd like to get into your pants, so it's harder
to understand why it upsets us if a guy says this to us. Break the

habit of writing off what you don't understand. Next time she's upset about something you see as trivial, nicely (force yourself!) ask her to explain what she's feeling and why it's important. Just because you don't understand something at face value, doesn't mean she's wrong! Understand and show compassion.

FROM DEFENSE TO OFFENSE

It's counterproductive to take what we say or do personally. If we don't take your advice, we still value you. If we do something ourselves, we still need you. Women complain about how defensive you get if we disagree with you. It causes more static. Don't be so defensive. Cheyna said:

> *Ray jokes about being "the man" but I know he's serious. When he offers to help me do something, he acts insulted if I do it myself. I'm starting to become self-sufficient and it feels good. I'm sure he does some things much better than me but how can I learn if he does everything for me? I think he's the best and I look up to him as a man. He doesn't believe me. If I don't treat him as the God all-knowing man, he thinks I don't have confidence in his abilities. It's ridiculous. We have to boost men's egos like they're children.*

Some of your defensiveness starts in childhood. I don't want to get too psychological, but you've all been influenced to a degree by your relationship with Mom. Your attitude toward women was shaped in part by her. If she scolded you a lot, you may still be a defensive little boy when you interpret things we say or do as criticism. We're not criticizing you if we make suggestions. We don't see you with major shortcomings because we air a grievance. We still love you and respect your ability when we challenge something you do. Remember—if we didn't like you so much, most of what we chide you about wouldn't matter to us.

LYING—THE NUMBER ONE COMPLAINT FROM WOMEN

The women I interviewed consistently had stories of men who lied to them. Lying comes in many varieties. One is a type of guy that I warn women about in *All Men Are Jerks Until Proven Otherwise*.

Some men have learned how to play women. They can cause a lot of the damage in women that translates into future reactions that you hate. Some of you have big egos, especially in larger cities, where the proportion of men to women is way in your favor. I find that in New York. You see women as toys to play with at your will. We spoil you in an effort to have a man and you have fun at our expense. Playing up to a woman you're really not interested in is deception, and isn't nice. Marcia complained:

> I recently met Mack. Our first date was lovely. We had so much in common. He expressed joy in meeting me and was very romantic. He kissed me a few times gently, but I let him know I wanted to take it slow. He respected that. He talked about things he'd like to share with me on future dates. When he walked me home, he held my hand and gently kissed me. Later that night I got an e-mail from Mack, saying how he was still on air from our interaction and still had my scent on his hands, from the perfume on my arms. He added that he couldn't wait to cuddle with me. I never heard from him again. After ten days, I e-mailed him, asking what happened. He wrote back saying that he'd met a woman he was compatible with, and wished me good luck. I'm flabbergasted. Why send the e-mail after if we weren't compatible? We seemed to be on our date. Even though nothing went down that night, I feel violated.

Too many women complained about meeting someone they liked, being swept off their feet, and then getting discarded like a broken toy. Me too. And I'm not talking about men who get sex and leave, which is also very wrong if you've led her to believe you like her for more than that. I mean guys that lead women on initially, when they know they're really not into her. The lack of respect for a woman's feelings if you toy with her for your own amusement or ego is shameful. Sorry guys, but this is one issue that I don't love you for. Dating lots of women isn't a sport, unless you tell her she's just your fox for the night. I'm much less open with men because of this behavior. It's what motivated me to write *All Men Are Jerks Until Proven Otherwise*. I know that most of you don't fall into this category if you're reading this book. But some men will read it to get better at playing women.

Please don't do that, no matter how easy it is and how much it builds your ego. What goes around does come around. I don't believe that guys who do that are sincerely happy. When you need to hurt others to make yourself feel good, it's a bad kind of good.

Many of you justify not always telling the truth. We can push you to lie, you say. If we look at you after a date with that "Please say you'll call me" look in our eyes, it's hard not to say "I'll call," even if you won't. Although it's more awkward on the spot, a generic statement such as "It was nice seeing you" lets us know not to sit by the phone waiting for your call. Yes, guys, many of us stay home and available in case you call. Spare us!

We push you to lie by making it unpleasant to tell the truth. If our reaction to what you tell us is over the top, lying seems easier. Brian said, "Debbie thinks my friend Theo is a bad influence. When I see him she gives me a cold shoulder afterward and withholds sex. So I say I did something else." Ryan added, "Hallie hates me drinking with my college buddies. When I tell the truth she goes off on me. It's easier to lie." Establish new boundaries. Although we may ask for it, the bottom line is lying kills trust in a relationship. Tell her nicely but straightforwardly why you feel a need to lie; that you'll tell the truth and walk out of the room if she reacts unfairly.

Satisfying Her Need for Attention

We drive you crazy with our need for attention. You ask all the time why women need so much. If you understand that it's quality time we need, and give us some, you'll spend less time trying to please us. We bug you for what we see as attention because we're afraid of losing you and see a lack of attention as a lack of interest. That's why small connections are so important. Fear of you leaving can be our equivalent of your fear of losing a good job. If you're the achievement and you leave, her life may seem lost.

Most of you have several things in your life of significant importance. For many of us, our original program says you're the one and only. You don't always make us your top priority and we hate that! While we need to accept you can't be our whole life and are entitled to space, we'd feel more secure with consistent reminders that we're *very* special to you; that you're proud of us; that you think of us often. Without them, we lose that connection we need. Making a little time for us each day softens rough spots. Here are more things you can do that help satisfy our needs. They're fun for you, too, if you allow them to be! Find little things that nurture our need to connect. The rewards of a satisfied woman are great!

MAKE TIME FOR HER

If you don't want to share quality time, why be there at all? To get cleaning, cooking, and sex? We can feel like a housekeeper or prostitute. Figure out why you give time to others but can't find energy to do things with her. If you purposely withhold attention because the need for it annoys you, please reconsider. Quality time with the woman you care about can give you joy too. Make a conscious effort to have quality time with your partner every day if you live together, even if it's ten minutes of snuggling before going to sleep. A connection every day goes a long way. Take a walk together after dinner. Have a laugh at the supermarket. Clean or wash the car together. Have fun doing whatever you do together. Take a class. Join a club. Support a candidate. Plan a getaway. Tickle. Be goofy.

♡ **Connection Tip**

Thank her for being the special woman she is—regularly. Thank her for specific things she does too.

DON'T TAKE HER FOR GRANTED

If you're just dating, it can be easier—you have less opportunity to take each other for granted. Quality time together helps keep your relationship off of autopilot. When you've been together for some time, things can get stale. That's not necessary! We get complacent because we're comfortable together. We forget to say "I love you" or even "Have a nice day." Never take your partner for granted! Treat her the way you'd like to be treated and she'll probably reciprocate. Regularly show appreciation for who she is and what she does. Stay conscious of the good things she brings to your life. Express your feelings. Give kisses and hugs. Don't let them become a habit. That's a form of taking for granted. If you say or do it, please mean it. Don't be insincere to placate her! If you care, show her!

TREAT HER AS YOU DID WHEN YOU FIRST MET

I agree with your gripes about us slacking on our appearance. Women admit that when they're in a long-term relationship, they stop wearing makeup and worrying about what to wear. Change that without complaining. I know you can't do it all the time but find ways to be spontaneously romantic. Make love to your partner like she's your one and only. No matter how long you've been together, always see her as your lover. It's easy to take her for granted. Remember why you fell for her. And reciprocate with attention to your own grooming (see Chapter 8). Compliment her when she makes an effort to look good. Make her want to keep her appearance up for you!

RECAPTURE OR MAINTAIN THE PASSION

Use the ideas in this book to connect with her. Most women will make more of an effort to look good and please you if you do. Bring her a dozen roses for no reason or take her to a romantic dinner and she'll try harder to please you. Bring out the special woman in her by treating her like a special woman! Cook her dinner. Bathe her in bubbles. Send notes or call her in anticipation. Treat her as a woman, not just a sex partner. Romance works wonders (more in Chapter 9).

REGULARLY MAKE SPECIAL DATES WITH YOUR PARTNER

No matter how long you've been together, ask her out like you just started dating. Relationships can get sweeter with time if you want them to. Treat her as you would a new woman in your life. It's fun! Plan an evening that she'd like and surprise her. Do things that you know she'll like, even if going to the theater or to a lecture isn't your idea of a great date. Let her do it for you the next month. The most important thing is spending quality time together. Bernie said:

I've been with my girlfriend for three years but I still love to make her feel special. I love planning a special evening out and I tell her in advance that we're having a special night on, let's say, Friday. I make her feel special all day. I call her at work and let her know I'm looking forward to our time out. I tell her how terrific she is and why I want to make her happy when we do things. By the time we go she's all excited, like she was when we first started dating. You've always got to treat your woman like she's special because she is, isn't she? If you don't think so, why are you with her?

CREATE RITUALS THAT INVOLVE SHARING TIME

No matter how busy you are, make time. Set one night a week aside to watch videos in bed. Go for a special brunch every other Sunday. Read the paper in bed together. Make her breakfast. Hold her hand when you go out. My parents were married for over fifty years and still lovingly held hands, still kissed because they wanted to, and still got excited about getting in the car and going on an overnight adventure. I'm very blessed that I had such good role models for how a healthy, loving relationship can sustain and grow for so many years. You need to nurture your partner and the love you feel. If she means enough to you, it should be your pleasure. You just need to get the hang of it.

APPEAR TO BE SPONTANEOUS IN YOUR EXPRESSIONS OF CARING

Not only do we want time, we want to know you want it too. We want "show and tells" that say you care. Chaz said if his wife wants something, she should spell it out and he'll put it in his diary. He said, "If she wants flowers I can put it on my to-do list every week. She says she doesn't want them that way. It should be spontaneous if I love her. Of course I'd do it because I love her. What do women want?" We don't want you to do things by rote! We'd like to feel you bought flowers because you got an urge to please—you thought about her and were motivated to do something special. Doing something small but special for your partner is something to enjoy getting into the habit of doing—just don't use the word *habit* in front of her!

Leave Your Mother Home

NEVER compare your partner to your mother! It can cause big problems if she's sensitive. If you're close with mom, jealousy can intrude. You may spend more time catering to the first woman in your life than she feels is appropriate. Your mate wants to be your top priority, so resentment can brew from giving mom too much attention or if she thinks you expect her to follow in mom's footsteps. You may not realize how many times you bring up how mom did things, thinking you're being helpful with constructive suggestions. But it most likely won't be welcome. A suggestion is fine once in a while. See how she responds; she may not mind. But since she wants to be your number one woman, her way should be tops in your book. Be sensitive to this.

Balance Work and Play

Many of you say you work long hours out of responsibility as the provider. But being gone a lot and not being all there at home can kill a relationship. You call her unsupportive if she complains. Are you convinced that you're sacrificing for her? Listen to what she says. Your ambition is what drives you, not her. If your partner complains you're working too much, she doesn't want you to. Some of you work to satisfy your ego as a good provider. But working all the time doesn't make you a good partner. If your mate asks you to choose between her or your job, you're probably compulsively working. Be careful—a job isn't worth a good partner. Too many of you regret, too late, not cutting back on your work time to allow more time for fun and enjoying your partner. Avoid this mistake. Leave work at work. If necessary, ask for thirty minutes of peace when you get home to unwind and make a transition from work to home.

It's unfair to expect you to put everything aside, but we can compromise. Set boundaries but don't take us for granted. Everything else can't come first if you want a relationship with a happy woman. Show respect and consideration. Let her know if you'll be late. Value her time and spending time with her. Little things can bring big rewards!

Connection Tip

If she's someone who can't make up her mind easily, try offering her two choices. "Where do you want to eat? How about the diner or Italian restaurant?" Pull a decision from there.

What's Really on the Minds of Women?

You complain women can't make up their minds. Why do we waiver back and forth when making decisions? Many of us haven't been taught to think for ourselves. We're concerned about what everyone wants, so making choices has more variables than yours. Believe me, it's not easy to make a decision for ourselves when we're trying to please others.

MAKE UP YOUR MIND!

Why we have a hard time making up our minds is actually very simple. We have conflicts between what we actually want and what we think you'll want us to choose. Our program to be nice provokes guilt if we don't do the right thing. You make decisions based on what you'd like. We weigh what others would want too. We'll agree to things because we don't want to displease you. Paulette was happy hearing she wasn't alone:

> I always have a tug of war with myself about what I'd like to do and whats gets shoved on me. I have a wonderful boyfriend who said we could get married if it's important to me. It's important to my mother. She expects me to get married. I'm happy living with him for now. I make many choices based on what's expected of me, which I hate. My boyfriend gets impatient when I can't make simple decisions. Where do I want to eat? I wonder where he wants to eat. It's those old worries about not pleasing your man. I don't want to decide something he won't like. Yet I make decisions about important policies at work with no problem. What's best for my company is easy. What I want is open-ended.

Our program translates "What do you want?" into "What would he like me to do?" We worry too much about making a decision that pleases you, and instead, we annoy you! It all boils down to insecurity. Since many of us don't think we deserve what we want, we try to please you so you'll want us.

Reading Our Minds?

You say that trying to find out what we want is a losing battle. We throw mixed signals because we're not comfortable being direct. We circumvent and hope you love us enough to know. Since we use intuition, we assume you can read our minds. Most of you complain that you can't.

We're not always good at accepting kindness or gifts. Our program is for giving, so it's hard to receive. But don't always take what we say literally. If she says "You don't have to be at my presentation. It won't interest you," be there, or she may be devastated! We say things to let you off the hook because of our guilt program (a big bug in our hard drives). We want you to care enough to want to do what's important to us. If she says "I'm too old for birthday gifts. Don't waste money—I don't need anything." Ha! Get something nice to prove her wrong—a "show and tell" that you don't think she's old *and* she deserves it. If she says it's unnecessary to do something that's special to her, she wants it. Giving her something nice is always good.

We say things we don't mean out of insecurity—we feel guilty asking for what we truly want. "You don't have to be home when I return from my trip." Ha! If you thrive on resentment don't be there. "Don't bring a gift from your trip." Double Ha! Listen only if you don't care about sex. If she points out how expensive something is that she loves, she wants you to think she's worth the expense. "Here's the ring as a token of how special you are." Have compassion, guys; learn to read our signals!

Giving Satisfying Support

You're known for helping. That's fine if it's help we'd like. Do you feel responsible for "helping" her to be a better person? Get over it! While you complain she tells you what to do, many of you also do that, under the guise of "helping." Unwanted suggestions to "improve" are harmful to a relationship.

Support vs. Unwanted Solutions

When something bothers you, you either take care of it or try not to think about it. We like to get it off our chests verbally. Your achievement program pushes you to suggest what to do about it. If you can't think of something constructive to say, you often ignore us. We don't like either! There's a difference between support and unsolicited directions. Here are some common differences between what men and women need that causes static in our interactions. These aren't new to most of you but I must emphasize them.

+ If something bothers you, you seek space and want to be alone. We seek comfort with someone.

+ You prefer to go into yourself and not talk. We want to discuss it and get consolation.

+ When we complain, we want supportive words or sympathy. You tend to give a practical suggestion or say nothing, which upsets us.

+ You're programmed to find solutions. We're programmed to seek support and empathy. We need to vent, and crave a sympathetic ear to dump on, not instructions.

Don't take it personally if she doesn't want to hear your assessment of her problem. We need you to listen and give comfort. I know we often go on and on—bear with us. It's our way of handling problems. Don't tell her what to do. Instead, offer compassion and encouragement. Acknowledge her right to whatever emotions come out of a situation—whether she's angry, hurt, tired, or fed up. Don't make light of it or say it's not important. It is to her. Offer sympathy, even if you think she's silly to feel as she does. She's entitled to her feelings.

Constructive Help

You often rush to show your talents and prove what a man you are. This can come across as patronizing if she didn't ask for it—like you think you're better or smarter or that she's not capable. She may feel treated like a little girl. If you want to help, support her. If she makes a mistake, don't tell her what she should have done. Instead, play up her good qualities—reinforce her abilities if it's a work-related problem, or give compliments if she's been offended. That's all many of us want. We don't need berating. We do that enough to ourselves. Comfort her with hugs, kind words, and a shoulder to cry on. Don't say what you'd have done. Hugs work better!

Encourage our endeavors. Don't be scared of losing us. Some of you discourage our dreams or sabotage our self-improvement because you're afraid we'll leave. We need your support and approval. We have a right to grow as women. Cheer us on if we go back to school or risk a career change. Some of you try keeping our confidence level low so we'll have to stay. You don't want us that way! A happier woman is a healthier partner. If we love you, why should we leave? If you know why, work on what you think your problem is—make yourself a healthier and more supportive partner.

PMS: Fact or Excuse?

You complain about dealing with our PMS. Until you've experienced it, you can't imagine how it feels to go through body changes that vary from insignificant to debilitating every month for a large part of adulthood. Not every woman gets the symptoms you associate with it—the grouchy, irrational mood swings many of us put you through each month. I want you to step back from your annoyance and jokes about PMS and try to understand the discomfort many of us endure. Test your compassion because we need it here.

THE LOWDOWN ON PMS

Do you want to make us angry? Then go ahead, ask: "Are you PMSing?" Some of you have an annoying habit of assuming that if we lose our tempers or are in a bad mood, it's our "time of the month." We get upset other times too! I see red if you assume I'm not letting you get away with something because of PMS, since I don't get those mood swings. I once had a fight with a boyfriend who smugly stated, "All women get PMS moods." When I said, "not me!" he arrogantly said that while he hadn't seen it, he was sure I did because all women do. There's a difference between PMS mood swings and the body changes women get monthly.

★ *PMS Relief*

When you know she's PMSing, bring something to cheer her up— a nice lotion, a small sweet treat, or whatever she might like.

So what exactly is PMS? It stands for pre-menstrual syndrome. Our bodies go through hormonal changes each month before our period. All women have PMS, but not all of us have the mood swings. Our bodies also get bloated, our breasts get sore, and we suffer other annoyances. Many women gain about three pounds for a few days and get cravings for salty foods and sweets. But PMS can have a serious effect on the behavior of many women. I'll let some describe it for you. How would you like to go through this kind of discomfort every month? Julie feels most of you don't want to know about PMS. She explained:

I don't think men understand that PMS can start during ovulation and last ten days—that it's a physical thing, caused by a change in hormones, that we have no control over. I get extremely sensitive and sometimes want to cry all day. I could have a day where you'd say "Hi Julie" and I'd burst into tears. Sometimes I look at myself and laugh—I'm sitting and crying for no reason. I think "what the F am I crying about?" A week before my period I put on weight, feel bloated, get sensitive and irritable. It affects my work. I easily misconstrue things and get angry at myself the next day. PMS is a pain in my ass.

Teri gave her feeling:

For three to five days every month I alternate between a very miserable, weepy mood and anger. Any little thing makes me go into a rage. I make nasty comments without knowing where they came from. There's usually nothing going on to cause this. I deny it and tell myself to snap out of it but can't. It's often scary because I get irrational—run off crying or scream at someone and not know why.

It's especially bad during stressful times. I keep thinking there must be a reason for it but there's not.

And Florence:

Guys make jokes about PMS but can't begin to understand what it's like to dread living through almost a week every month. Before my period I get moody. My body gets bloated, my breasts are sore. Sometimes I get depressed and too tired to do anything. I want to leave work. Everything and everyone bothers me. It feels like I'm cracking up. Then some guy gives me a "Do you have PMS, yuk, yuk?" line—I want to kill him. Guys should thank God they don't get this. I feel totally out of control. Oh, did I mention the painful cramps for three days? Guys need to know it's no laughing matter.

We can't control PMS. There's no cure. Each month most of us suffer at least some of the symptoms. Some of you act as though it's our fault or we could do something if we wanted. Women have said it's scary knowing they may say or do things during this time and have little control over it.

GETTING THROUGH PMS

So what do you do when you see signs of PMS besides run? Show compassion. As much as you don't like us having it, we like it less. It's unpleasant so please be patient! You've said the best way to handle our PMS is to give us lots of space. Myrna said, "I tell my husband and kids it's PMS time. They know that means to leave me alone as much as possible if they know what's good for them."

Bob and his girlfriend developed rules for PMS week. "Carla's like another person but I know she can't help it. We make decisions about how I should respond when she's PMSing. Sometimes I have to leave her alone. Sometimes she needs hugs. We've discussed it so there's no surprises." Talk to your partner when she doesn't have it and ask what she'd like you to do during PMS. Julie advises, "If your partner has PMS, tread gently and keep a smile on your face. Be sensitive."

4

SECURITY GLITCHES:
WHY WE CRASH WITHOUT REASSURANCE

Your partner walks in looking pretty but you're busy and say nothing. She asks, "How does this dress look on me?" "Good," you respond as you work on your project. She startles you when she complains that you don't like her dress. "Why do you think that?" you ask. "Because you only said 'good,'" she cries. You think for a minute and say, "You look very, very good," thinking that she'll understand you love it. But instead she leaves the room crying that you never say anything nice and you don't love her. What did she expect? You complimented. Of course you love her. How are you supposed to show it? By constantly saying "I love you?" By kissing up to her all the time? No way! You're angry as you think, "Why do women need so damn much reassurance!" ～

This chapter explains why and illustrates where compassion is most needed. You complain we can be totally insecure. We need too many expressions of feelings and compliments. We ask questions about our looks that can provoke trouble no matter what you say. You're right—many of us are guilty as charged. Dealing with our insecurity is hard but we have a harder time dealing with ourselves. Put yourselves in our shoes to understand where our programs come from. Compassion will be greatly appreciated.

Fragile Self-Esteem
Women get judged on many levels, from all directions. As girls we're

programmed to look good and act nice so people like us. Teachers favor the prettiest and most acquiescent girls. We learn that the better we come across, the more we get. By puberty, we've honed our skills for being as appealing as possible to the opposite sex. It becomes the biggest factor for achieving goals.

HANDICAPPED BY JUDGMENTS

I got a message at a young age that if I didn't watch my weight, I wouldn't get a boyfriend. I wasn't fat but not being petite or thin made me feel inferior—even before I noticed boys. The most popular girls were the smallest. I liked my looks but my few extra pounds felt like a handicap. Boys with my equivalent body type were just considered normal.

When I was fifteen, a guy said that with my shape and face, I'd be a knock out, IF I lost a few pounds. That statement cut into my self-esteem and hurt me into adulthood. Looking back, I'm angry at his audacity. He was slovenly with a big belly, yet criticized me! But he got girlfriends with no problem. A woman with parallel looks wouldn't have gotten many dates. Many women settle for any old schlep, just to have the relationship we think we need.

Pressure to look good if we want to be liked is something many of you can't comprehend. I asked women what they believed to be contributing factors to insecurity in themselves and other women. Some responses were:

> **Mary (age 18):** It's probably due in part to the images portrayed in Hollywood and the media at large. I also think it's because women are so often critiqued solely on the basis of their looks. Many parents encourage this focus on physical appearance in their daughters, which can be damaging, especially in those self-conscious teenage years.

> **Yvonne (age 41):** I feel terrible because so many men are into physical appearances. They want a model-like woman. Some men we've dated make us feel insecure.

> **Nora (age 34):** We are constantly told by the media, our peers, etc. that we are supposed to be ways that mostly don't come

naturally to us. Also many woman have had bad relationships with their parents and are plagued by negative voices.

Amy (age 26): Upbringing—parents bringing us up without adequate praise; media portrayal of a supermodel body as the most desirable. If we don't feel pretty or sexy and men don't pay attention to us, it eats away at self-confidence.

Mandi (age 19): We can't live up to society's standards.

Lee (age 42): From the cradle to the corporate world we are second-class citizens. We get too tired to fight for something different.

Gia (age 55): As I get older, I feel pressure to hide my age. I've never felt I could be as good as was expected but aging makes it worse. Youth is heralded in woman. I need my husband to reassure me that he's not going to leave me for a younger woman.

Adria (age 29): We're not brought up with confidence and individuality.

Jackie (age 38): Women compete with each other for attention. I've never felt secure around attractive women, though I look good. I worry about falling short in a comparison. Beautiful women seem to have it made. The rest of us settle.

Jenna (age 23): There are beautiful women out there. We want to know that, to our man, we are the most beautiful woman in the world . . . we are the smartest, sweetest, best cook, best lover, etc. We are competitive beings.

Judy (age 41): We only got the vote during the twentieth century!

Carrie (age 35): When I was a kid, being smart made my self-esteem lower. The pretty, silly girls got the attention. I always felt I had to be low-key about my abilities and play up my looks. I don't know who I am if I can't take pride in my intelligence.

We judge ourselves more than you judge us, and can be our own worst critics, chipping away at our fragile sense of self. Pressure to look good starts with friends. We learn young to compete for your attention and jealousy results. Girls get jealous of friends who have boyfriends when they don't, and those with nicer bodies, hair, clothing, etc. Many of us still do it. We compliment each other with negatives—"I wish I had your body." "I'd kill to have hair like yours." Some of you ask if we're more concerned about our appearance for other women. Women can be their own worst enemies—nurturing each other's insecurity. Unless we develop real self-esteem, our worth is depends on your input.

 Romantic Tip

Compliment the parts of her body that you love when she's not asking. Follow that with some affection before she can refute you.

WHAT IS SELF-ESTEEM?

What's real self-esteem? I see it as unconditional self-approval—being comfortable in your own skin—what we think of ourselves, as imperfect and human. I had a boyfriend who described it as striving to be as perfect as possible. He was never happy with himself, or me. Perfect is impossible. Self-esteem is accepting *you* as is. It's okay to want to change things. I feel better when I take care of my health and body for me, not to attract you. Most women don't get it. If we set impossible standards, we'll never reach them. Becky wrote to me:

> I'm a successful designer but always worried about my looks. I'm considered attractive but past boyfriends always found something about my body that could be better. I worked out but it was never good enough. I was apologetic about my body with Rick when we first had sex. He reassured me but I didn't believe him. One day he put me in front of the mirror when we were both naked and pointed out everything he loved about me, which he said is what he sees when he looks at me. He then pointed to parts of his body that weren't perfect and asked if I was turned off. I got the message and

appreciate myself more and more. My self-esteem is growing. Bless Rick for his patience.

Self-esteem is what we think of ourselves but we're not programmed to think for ourselves. How can we have a positive self-image if what we think is secondary to your opinion? Compliments are like Band-Aids. Self-esteem goes up if you want us. It dissipates if you leave. Do you see why we need reassurance?

Our ultimate source of pressure is you! I asked both sexes to rate the importance of many qualities in the opposite sex. Women didn't minimize the importance of appearance, but most didn't give it nearly as much importance as you. The kind of person you are carried more weight in their attraction to a man. Man after man apologetically referred to himself as shallow as he acknowledged that looks weighed very heavily in deciding who to go out with. And you wonder why we're so insecure about our looks?

Distorted Images

People have said that low self-esteem is like an epidemic among women. A large percentage of us find fault with at least some aspect of our appearance. Our need to be perfect enables us to see teeny flaws that you'd never notice. We magnify and stress over them. And we hate ourselves for having them.

I rarely meet women who are completely happy with their looks. Those with stunning bodies show me an extra quarter of a pound they're convinced needs to go. You'd be amazed if you could see us in the distorted mirrors, created by our minds, that many of us see ourselves in—we gain weight and have flaws you won't see. In my workshops, women use "unattractive" or "fat" to describe themselves. Few are accurate. We're obsessed with being perfect. Gwen, a slender size six, justified:

I know I'm slim but you haven't seen my stomach and thighs. I don't get complaints from men but I'm sure they're being polite. I see flab in my stomach. My thighs aren't firm enough. I don't want a man to leave me because my body's not perfect. These days I never let a boyfriend see me fully naked. I wear sexy lingerie and make sure the lights are out before we have sex. Why take chances on being rejected?

Your fixation on our bodies creates stress about weight. Many of you admitted pushing at least one girlfriend to diet. It makes us feel awful. *You* eat more without gaining and don't understand how tough it can be to lose weight under pressure. I had a boyfriend push me to lose a few pounds. But when I asked to stop eating out so much, he told me to go to the gym more. He couldn't relate—I had to eat less to maintain my weight but he refused to accept that. You're notorious for sarcastic comments, pushing us to the gym, or trying to control our eating. Then you bristle at our insecurity. Criticism from you hurts. We put ourselves down enough. I tell women they can't change you—the same goes for you. Lighten up, guys. Pushing us to lose weight won't help. Supporting us can.

Are you aware of how much people pick on our appearance? I've gained a few pounds on vacation and gotten comments. Few acknowledged my losing them. Men don't need as much reassurance. John said, "[Compliments] should be gravy, not expected. I can go for months without one without realizing I have until one comes along . . . I'm happy without them and even happier when I get one." Those of you who don't need positive words are lucky. You're not self-conscious. People don't put you down as much. You don't care if someone notices a haircut or new shirt. We assume disapproval if you say nothing. Dawn said:

> *I'd be fine if I didn't have to see people. I look in the mirror in the morning and like what I see. My ego can be deflated by lunchtime. Someone may ask why I got my hair cut—it looked better before. I can have facial lines pointed out with recommendations for getting rid of them. A friend may ask if I've gained a pound. I may meet my boyfriend for lunch who says nothing good, which worries me. People are stupid but I take it seriously.*

We need positive words but refuse to believe them. You can't tell us too many times that you love us or our looks. While we're dying for compliments, they're hard to accept. Only in the last few years have I been able to accept a compliment by just saying "thank you." Most of my life I put myself down in response to compliments, because I didn't believe them and I'd been taught that people like modest girls better.

If the fat talk drives you crazy, sit down with her when you're both in a good mood. Nicely, ask her to let you explain your feelings without interruption. Tell her how annoying it is; that you're happy with her or you wouldn't be there. Ask what you can do to help her feel better. Offer to exercise with her if that might help. Give her compliments and ask her to please try to accept that you're happy with her the way she is. Keep annoyance out of your voice, no matter how hard it is.

Getting older is another very sensitive issue. There's a double standard about aging. It adds character to *you*. Gray hair and lines make you distinguished/debonair. There are no sexy "older" words for us, so we fear you won't want us if we look older. It's changing (thanks to lovely ladies like Susan Sarandon and Jamie Lee Curtis), but many of us see aging as losing attractiveness. That's ridiculous. I know I'm better now than ever and date younger guys. Most women don't. Even many with great self-esteem still won't tell their age. More of you appreciate women who are older but the stigma is still there—another source of insecurity.

INDEPENDENT, SUCCESSFUL WOMEN = ATTRACTIVE OR THREATENING?

You say you're attracted to independent and successful women, but many of you can't handle it. I'm sure you find us attractive. We're low maintenance—sexy, stimulating, a challenge—able to give you space. But your program as provider/protector may not be as comfortable with a woman who takes care of herself. I should be a dream woman for many men. Guys lust after me but end up with the helpless maiden they complain is too needy. What a shame for both sexes.

Many of us know you get intimidated by a successful, confident, independent, and/or very smart woman. We've been taught these qualities make us seem "unfeminine" in some eyes, which doesn't motivate us to show them. We know how to play airhead. When we meet a guy we're not sure can handle a together woman, we keep it under wraps. I know loads of women who believe they have to "play the role" in order to not scare you off.

Men with money and powerful positions, even unattractive ones, get dates. Many women are attracted to money/power/success. But these qualities in a woman, even a very attractive one, usually don't get the same results. You say they can threaten your sense of self. Can you handle a woman who's more successful than you? Be honest. Would a woman who made more money or had a better job make you feel less of a man? You find independence and success attractive on one level. But a large number of you admitted you were insecure about a woman with a more successful career. Sam said it broke up his marriage:

> I was attracted to Janet because she was smart. I fell in love quickly and thought her career was wonderful. Her success was exciting. Our first years of marriage were happy and I accepted that she was vice president of a large corporation and made a lot more money. But as her career escalated faster than mine, our income gap got wider. I didn't feel like a man. Janet was low-key but wanted to spend her money—I didn't want her to. As the man, I wanted to pay for half of everything. But I couldn't afford what she wanted. She had a right to spend what she earned but it made me feel less of a man when she did. It killed our marriage. I admit, it was all me. I created the problem. Janet never understood why it bothered me every time she spent money. That macho bullshit is ingrained!

Men I date ask variations of "What's a woman like you doing with a man like me?" It's a quandary. Now that my career's doing well, it's hard to meet guys who aren't intimidated by what I do. I have a high-powered career but keep my personal life simple. In a relationship, I love being low-key and pampered and don't want to be in charge. But knowing I can take care of myself is enough to intimidate many of you. Other successful women agree. Yet many of you are attracted to us initially. Those of you not happy with your career may see us as reminders that you aren't where you want to be. You may like feeling needed and don't understand we do need you—in healthier ways.

Smart Answers to Those Dumb Questions

Why do we ask questions with no good answers? There are enough jokes around about the futility of answering questions like "Does this outfit make me look fat?" to ensure that every woman should have the message. Yet we continue to torment you and ourselves. Insecurity plays havoc with our thinking.

Do I Look Fat?	
DON'T SAY	DO SAY
No.	I love how you look.
Stop asking that.	Your curves are sexy.
I answered that yesterday.	No, you don't need to change.

The Questions

"Do I look fat?" Questions about our appearance, especially weight, put you in a lose/lose spot. There's rarely a satisfying answer yet we keep asking. Answering "yes" has obvious consequences. Saying "no" can lead to more lose/lose questions such as "Does my butt look big?" because we don't believe you. When we ask digging questions, we're hoping you'll find magic words to reassure us once and for all. They don't exist. Our insecurity makes us suspect even the sincerest compliments. John is frustrated by his wife's inability to lose the weight she's gained. He reassures her to no avail and finds the truth counterproductive, as she becomes more insecure and gains more weight. He said in frustration:

> Women have an ability to distort and warp reality in order to avoid confronting it. "Do these pants make me look fat?" No. Pants don't make you look fat, your big rolls of fat make you look fat. Her question should be "How good a job do these pants do to hide how fat I am?" I get this question more than once a week.

"How do I look?" questions can be easier to answer, but also require diplomacy. We grill you with "Do you like my new dress on me?" "Which shoes look better with this outfit?"—"Should I cut my hair?" Think before answering these often trick questions, unless you like the taste of your foot in your mouth. Avoid answers that lead to more questions. Do you think saying her dress makes her look thinner is good? She may follow with "Do I usually look fat?" Choose one pair of shoes—"Why don't you like the other?" Nancy admitted:

> I ask my husband questions about my looks all the time. It drives him mad but I can't stop. I look in the mirror and worry. So I ask him. He says nice things but I don't believe it. Yet I want to hear so I keep asking. I don't know what would satisfy me. I'm insecure and scared my husband will wake up one day, see what I see and leave. I wonder if I keep asking questions about my looks to test him, to make sure he sees I'm not perfect. It's a bad cycle. I ask, he answers, I don't believe him and ask again, and so on. I wish I could feel good about myself. I think I'm pushing him to say the negative things I believe. It's ridiculous that I ask and ask about the same things, knowing I won't accept his answer.

These questions are part of our reassurance game. I told you what we may see in the mirror. If we feel shame or doubt about our looks, we reach out for reassurance. But our low self-esteem prevents us from believing you. I must emphasize that not nearly all women are like this. Many ask questions to get legitimate input. It's quickly obvious whether your partner is one who wants an answer or one who needs reassurance. Don't lump us all together.

The Answers

What's the right answer for lose/lose questions? "I'm late for a meeting—must run" or changing the subject rarely works. I wish there were specific responses but each woman and question is different. Answers like "No, you don't look fat" or "Your dress is nice" are too generic. They sound as though you're giving lip service, without much thought. We want to know you've given your answer personal consideration. Guys, please understand how important your words are and use compassion in answering. When we ask "Do I look good/fat?" we already believe the worst and want you to change our minds.

Sometimes going into details helps. Tell us why you like our hair now *and* why you think we'd look good with it short too, including compliments. Specific reasons sound more truthful—"Your face is so pretty that short hair would accentuate it but your long hair is sexy—I enjoy playing with it." Pleading ignorance laced with compliments can work—"I know very little about putting outfits together. Your taste is much better than mine—you always look great. Both shoes are nice—it's hard for me to choose. I trust your taste." If you say, "I don't know" she'll interpret it as a negative or not caring.

Are you getting the picture? I'm being honest. If your woman asks lose/lose questions and responds badly to your answers, be evasive, plead ignorance, and give specific compliments. Giving details instead of saying "No, you don't look fat," will be taken more seriously—"Of course you don't look fat. That shirt is sexy on you" or "You look great. I like that color on you—that blouse is hot/pretty/stylish, etc." Learn to describe so you can give the best answers to lose/lose questions. But don't patronize her! Use nice words to say what you feel—compliment what you really like. Something in this vein that we do that's terribly unfair to you is putting you on the spot by using "If you loved me enough you would . . ." to manipulate you into doing what we want. For example, you can either go shopping with her to prove your love or have her accuse you of not loving her because you didn't buy into the game. Call her on it, nicely. Tell her the choices are an unfair attempt to get her way. You love her but shouldn't have to go shopping to prove it. Self-esteem is a long process—your patience, compassion, and reassurance help.

"WHAT ARE YOU THINKING?"

How often have you heard a version of: "You're quiet, what are you thinking about?" or "You have a funny look. What's the matter?" or "Is everything okay?" from your partner? We get paranoid. You may have indigestion and we may read your face as your wanting out of the relationship. Honest! Some of us get uptight about something being wrong if your attitude toward us isn't pure love and joy.

If we had our way, some of us would monitor your thinking all the time, to make sure everything is okay. We can be concerned your feelings have changed, that you're cheating, that you no longer find us attractive, or other things we conjure up. Our need to know your thoughts is unnecessary. We shouldn't be privy to everything in your head. It gets worse if you say, "Nothing is wrong" when something is wrong. We can't distinguish between what might affect us and indigestion, so we question *all* your funny looks. Be honest if you don't want to share your thoughts, but not with an attitude.

 Connection Tip

> After sex, trace her curves lightly with your fingertips. This maintains the connection and shows appreciation for her body.

Reassuring Our Insecurity

I'll repeat myself—showing compassion for our insecurity goes a long way. Patience now can result in more peace later. Reassurance helps us relax with fears of not being adequate or losing you. It CAN get better. When her insecurity surfaces, show love instead of annoyance for long-term results. Here are suggestions for making her feel better and relax more.

STOP EXPECTING WOMEN TO BE PERFECT CREATURES

Perfection isn't real. Take the pressure off for both her sake and yours. You're at least partially responsible for perpetuating the notion that we have to look and act as good as possible. Ian said, "Women are insecure big time. But who helped to make them that way—men!" Many of you put us on pedestals when you first meet us and then start chipping away at the base as you see our imperfections. That's not fair! Alyssa told a class:

> *Damon treated me great when we started dating. I felt good about myself. Then he slowly made what he called suggestions about changes he'd like in me. They felt like digs. He suggested I join a gym to firm up, and wear clothing to turn him on more. When I said I thought he liked my looks, he said he'd like it better if I improved. Improved! In whose opinion? I tried what he wanted but it felt lousy. I told Damon he should accept me*

as I was. He insisted he wanted his woman to be the best she could and I should want to please him. I felt like I'd never be good enough to please him and was insecure most of the time. He wasn't perfect yet I accepted him. Eventually he left me for a woman who was thinner. Why do men think they're entitled to perfection in us? They're not perfect.

Cut Her Slack

A large number of women complained about men who criticized their appearance in ways that made them feel that if they didn't lose weight, style their hair, dress differently, use make up, or cover aging they'd leave, or continue making us feel like mud. Trying to meet your often-unfair expectations stokes our insecurity. Losing weight isn't easy, especially under pressure. I always lose weight when I'm in a happy relationship with a guy who seems happy with me. Our bodies digest food differently when we're stressed. Loving support is the best way to facilitate our looking better. A renovation campaign won't get happy results. Emma said:

> *When I was with Glen, I used to almost starve myself to lose the weight he hated. I tried but rarely lost any. I'd be nervous about losing Glen and wouldn't eat all day. Then he'd put me down more and I'd eat a lot. I don't understand why I hardly lost weight when I'd barely eat for weeks at a time. After breaking up, I met Terry. He's much more complimentary and talks like he's happy with me as I am. I was on edge at first, waiting for criticism. Slowly I relaxed as I became convinced that Terry likes me the way I am. I can't figure out why but my body's gotten into much better shape lately. Without the pressure of losing weight to keep someone, the weight comes off!*

Help Her Relax with Her Body

It's hard if your partner gains weight. People say it's unsupportive to find her unattractive when she's heavier. I disagree. It's normal and I don't blame those of you who, like John earlier, find it hard to accept. Overweight isn't attractive to many of us. But we gain weight for reasons. Work with us to find the cause and encourage us to try counseling, a nutritionist, or getting more exercise together. Harassing us to lose it rarely works. It causes bad feelings that make some of us want to eat more. Most of us would love to lose weight and do feel bad if we gain a lot, whether you tell us or not. We have eyes. Support works better. When I broke up with my boyfriend who bugged me to no avail, I lost the weight without trying, when I relaxed.

Don't Take Your Problems out on Her

If you don't feel good about yourself, you may pick on your partner more. If you're not content with your life; if you feel low about your job or income; if you don't feel respected—you may view your partner more critically as a reflection of how you feel about yourself. You may not be able to control your job or other people, but you can try controlling her appearance in an attempt to have one source of pride. That's not fair. Work on you!

Accept That We're Human

Our appearance isn't the only area of unrealistic expectations. Some of you expect us to be perfect about hygiene and body functions. Have you any idea how hard it is to be consumed by needing to be "ladylike"—neat, clean, soft, "nice girls"? Things that are totally acceptable in you may be deemed unladylike in us. Natural body functions are looked down on in a woman. I don't want to gross you out, guys, but I'm going to help you face facts that you know but may prefer not to think about. Women sweat, have gas, and do other things that create odors. Sherri wrote, "Amos expects me to be sweet and clean. Yet *he* doesn't need to be. I get self-conscious if I'm anything less. Please tell men that we're human." Contrary to media images of odorless, noiseless beings, women have body functions similar to yours. Many of us go to great lengths to hide them. It takes its toll on us. Some women deny what's not considered feminine. I've heard them say they don't sweat—they "glow" or "radiate." Let's be real! We're human. But our fear of turning you off creates tremendous pressure. Please accept us in our human state.

Reassure Her That She's Okay as Is

Accept us with our glitches, imperfections, humanness, and all.

We need you to reinforce our feeling attractive, sexy, worthy, and special—for who we are. It's a shame we need so much reassurance, but we got rules laced with criticism as girls, making it hard to accept ourselves. "Be good." "Stay neat." "Watch your weight." Compliments and reassurance soothe old wounds. Let her know she makes you happy and what it is about her that you find special. It means a lot. A few loving words now and then keeps most of us content. It's not a terrible tradeoff and makes us feel better. Sheila elaborated:

> *I've agonized over why I need so much reinforcement from my boy-friend. Sometimes he says he loves me but I want to hear it much more often. I want to know he's thoroughly attracted to me and I'm the only woman for him. I have a powerful job and know men are attracted to me. But I become the little girl who was insecure and needed to be told that she's good enough when I'm with Harold. I've had therapy but can't kick this. Most of my friends are this way. What is it about us? Why can't knowing we're good already be enough? Why does it have to come from him to confirm what I sincerely do know?*

♡ **Connection Tip**

Kiss the body parts that she complains about. If she thinks her tummy is flabby, kiss her all over and tell her you love it. Use words like soft, cute, curvy, etc. about them.

ADD SOME WORDS TO YOUR ACTIONS

I had a boyfriend who never expressed compliments or feelings. It drove me crazy. His actions left little doubt that he cared, yet I needed verbal expression. I craved compliments, though his eyes spoke them. When I'd complain he'd remind me he said I was very pretty on our first date. Wasn't that enough? No, it wasn't. It didn't dampen my appreciation for how well he treated me, but words were important too. Even me, an enlightened woman with great confidence in my looks still needed words. I'd get angry at myself. We don't like needing to hear them but can't help it. I promise your tongue won't fall off from too many loving words. Ben learned how much good he was able to do when he loosened his tongue:

The more Favia asked, the more I withheld my feelings. I debated whether to stay with her—she seemed so insecure. She's a beautiful woman—I didn't understand why I needed to keep telling her. When we were with her family, I did what you suggested—watched her with her father. She acted nervous about wanting to please him. I was surprised how he criticized her. He spoke positively to her brother but nitpicked Favia. Afterward I asked how her father treated her growing up. She said he found fault with whatever she did. Nothing was good enough in his eyes. You were right. A woman's insecurity can come from her father. Now I understand and show compassion. I let her know how I feel more often. What a change in Favia. She's more relaxed. I couldn't do it before—I thought it was dumb. Now I actually enjoy making her happy this way. Who'd of thought that?

Say the Nice Things You Feel

You may not realize how much time we spend preparing to go out. If you don't notice it, we feel let down. Others can compliment us, but until you do, many of us don't feel validated. I can look in the mirror and know I look hot but if my guy doesn't say something, I feel gypped. Give us what we need! Say what you feel, even if you think it's dumb. Try more generic statements like "It's great to see you" when you arrive or "I enjoy being with you" if you're having fun. It's no big deal and we love hearing it. Let's face it. Many of us would be thrilled with any expression. Don't fake it but if you feel good about your partner, find comfortable words to let her know once in a while.

Think the World of Her and Let Her Know It

"I think, therefore I am" (René Descartes). When you treat her as though you think highly of her, chances are she'll live up to your expectations. If you focus on her shortcomings, she can end up bitter and continue living up to your negative thoughts. Get in the habit of expressing appreciation for her. Regularly tell her that you love and appreciate her essence—who she is. Give her hugs while saying how much she means to you. Reinforce the beauty in her and she'll get more beautiful! Maximize her good qualities and she'll get even better!

5 EMOTIONS CRASH MY HARD DRIVE!
EMOTIONAL INCOMPATIBILITIES

You like your new girlfriend. She has all the qualities you've wanted in a woman. You spend more time together. Things heat up. As she begins to feel incredibly good to be with, memories of your last relationships haunt you. It took a long time to get over the last one. Suddenly you're hesitant to enjoy your new lady too much. What if she hurts you too? You cool down a bit. She notices and asks why. Of course you can't tell her. It's better to play it safe. So you dodge her questions and get cooler. All of a sudden things aren't the same between you. She's on your case and you're avoiding her. She says you're heartless and have no feelings. The problem is you have too many and can't cope with them. You wonder why you can't get it right in a relationship. Why can't women leave the feelings out of it and just have fun! Yet you ask yourself, *Why do I feel so lousy about pulling away from her? Why can't I figure this out?* ∾

Welcome to "Save Your Life 101." This is the longest chapter, since developing your emotional well-being is critical to a relationship. Absorb its content—you'll get along better and have fewer problems with us. This chapter is the springboard for a great relationship. To a degree, most problems are related to emotional responses. Learning to flex the muscles of your heart by stretching the walls that hold your feelings together, even just a little, will enable you to be a stronger man. I don't recommend making serious changes *for* a woman, unless the relationship is abusive. Change benefits **you**! It makes you a stronger man by putting you in control of yourself and how you respond to your emotions. You'll have a happier partner along with it. But do it for you!

Are we really so different when it comes to our emotions? Not from what you've told me. We all know how it feels to be hurt. Most of us have experienced some level of a broken heart and know it doesn't feel good. Men and women experience similar emotions. It's how we handle or perceive them that is different.

Understanding Our Emotional Responses

You complain we're much too emotional. Many of us live and breathe by our hearts. We pour emotions out while you keep them to yourselves. If we want to know what you're feeling and you won't let us in, we get even more emotional, which shuts you down more.

Our Upbringing

Although differences in the genetic makeup of males and females exist, my theory is that women are more emotional because we're conditioned to use emotions in childhood. Our "Nagging 101" classes begin early. Whining/crying doesn't work for boys. Girls conversely are shown if they get emotional, they can get what they want. A girl cries and gets a cookie. A boy cries and gets rejection—"Take it like a man." You get approval when you keep emotions to yourself. These formative messages have a profound effect on how we handle emotional issues.

As girls we learned that emotions are a tool for getting our way. If Dad said "no" and we nagged enough, it changed to "yes." When we wanted something and whined, adults gave in. We manipulated with tears and emotional maneuvers. That didn't work for you. As adults, we continue using tears for leverage while you continue stifling emotions. Playing people with emotions is so ingrained in our survival skills that we're not always aware we do it. Most of us still haven't figured out that it doesn't work. Liz said:

> I've always used tears to get my way. I even learned to fake them as
> a teen and continued using them to soften men. As I got older, my
> emotional outbursts didn't go over well with the men I dated. Some

gave in to me for a while. Some bolted. When I met Steve, I saw him as someone I could spend my life with and used my usual ways to get around things I didn't like. He stopped me in my tracks and asked what I was trying to accomplish. Steve was falling in love with me but getting turned off by my manipulating him with emotions. He assured me we'd stand a better chance of a long-term relationship if I tried honest communication instead. It's been hard to stop since it was second nature but Steve points it out to me when I backslide. Thank God I found a man who wasn't afraid to tell me the truth. Who knows how many men I lost in the past because of it?

I used to manipulate with emotions as a kid, and continued until I finally paid attention to the tone in my voice when I wasn't getting my way. I got nauseated. My voice was disgustingly whiny. It was so much a part of my makeup that I'd never been aware of that tone before. Needless to say I've made an all-out effort to change. I still use the whiny tone when I'm really upset but I control it most of the time. Many women can't.

♡ *Connection Tip*

When she's working at a computer, washing dishes, or engaged in something else, come up from behind and gently nuzzle/kiss her neck.

Do you still wonder why we can't break the habit of using emotions when we want something, and why you may not feel comfortable expressing them? It's hard to stop lifelong programs. Tough little boys grow into tough, self-sufficient, unemotional men. Delicate, whining girls grow into nagging, emotional women. We see over and over that it doesn't work for either sex but don't know what to do. Perhaps understanding where these patterns come from will enable you to be a little more patient with us.

ANGRY WOMEN

Anger is a big catalyst for our emotions. If you won't give us what we think you should, we get frustrated, then angry. Emotional outbursts can be the result of repressed feelings. When you express dissatisfaction, it's considered giving your opinion. When we express it, we may get negative reactions. We're programmed to be nice, quiet, and keep opinions to ourselves. We're good girls—until anger peaks.

Women can have a lot of suppressed anger. We get unwanted sexual advances; we earn lower salaries; we frequently experience double standards. We also have fewer acceptable outlets for our rage and stifle it a lot. We may reach our limit over a silly annoyance. Previous anger can pour into a response we dish at you, like a dam bursting. Understanding why we get angry is the key to not losing it with us. We need a loving response. Telling us to calm down, getting angry back, etc. fuels it more. Compassion works. Sue said:

> *So much made me angry growing up. My brothers had much more freedom than I did. I was supposed to be the good one. I had to watch them from the sidelines, having fun doing what I wished to do. It was unfair but I wasn't allowed to complain. If I told my grandma, she said that's how it was for girls. As I got older, I dated many men who treated me like a piece of meat, which made me angry. My friends and I complained but that made us angrier. Last week my husband and I were getting ready for a party and he asked me to wear my sexy red dress. I became a raving lunatic. All the memories of the past were in my rantings about not being a piece of meat or having to please him with my dress. Poor Jon. He had no idea of where all the anger directed toward his simple request came from.*

Men have more action-oriented outlets for anger—you break things, yell at people, punch a wall. If you curse and break things in anger, people accept it as normal for guys. These responses are considered unladylike so we circumvent anger by getting resentful, complaining, and throwing blame at others. We need to release it. Mary wrote:

> *Some of your outlets are healthy ones we could stand to learn from (being more confrontational/less back-stabbing). Some are F-ing stupid (punching in a windshield or getting obliviously strung out on drugs or drinking). When we're told to be good girls and not express ourselves, we hold our anger until we reach our boiling point.*

Coming Across as Heartless

How do you feel when we accuse you of having no feelings when you know you do? Since you don't show them our way, sometimes we say that you have no heart. Most of you said you have normal feelings but don't express them as well as you could. A majority of us believe you, but don't like your hiding them. We call you heartless creatures since you don't give us what we want.

Shutting Down

I must make you understand how devastating we find it when you go suddenly from being warm and loving to shutting down and getting cold. You rarely tell us why. The number one complaint I've had from women is that you can be warm and loving and then suddenly put up walls—big, high fortresses covered with icicles and gnarly barbs that hurt us if we try to get through. It can take a long time to recover from a man who shuts down after he's been warm and loving. Our trust can dissolve.

I guarantee that if we went cold on you with no explanation, you'd hate it too. But we rarely do, so you may not know what it feels like. If we go cold, there's usually more drama attached. We're also more likely to express the problem, since we want you to understand what's bothering us. You can get cold when something bothers you, which comes across as you not having feelings at all. It hurts. Try stepping into our shoes. Lanette said:

> My relationship with Bobby started in heaven. After four months in the best relationship of my life he suddenly changed. He got standoffish—practically stopped the affection he'd been pouring on me. I asked what was wrong and he gave the usual "nothing." Like I'm stupid! At first I panicked about losing him. I wondered if I knew him at all. I questioned my judgment in picking a man who'd hurt me by going cold. I wondered if he'd been using me. How can a man who said I mean the world to him turn off so quickly? Eventually he admitted he was scared because the relationship was going fast—at his doing! He wasn't sure how he felt. He'd been hurt by a girlfriend he trusted. We continued seeing each other but the trust was gone. I wondered what sort of monster

would do that to me. Friends said it's a guy thing. I can't believe that men don't know how this behavior hurts. How can they do it to someone they say they care for? It was a very painful time.

Raise your hand if you've done this! I bet many hands are up if you're honest. No matter how many times we experience it, we can't relate to how you can go inside yourself, go cold, or want nothing to do with us for a while if your feelings haven't changed. Some of you assured me that when you shut down, you mean no harm. It's your way of coping with something going on. Some of you said fear resulting from past experiences of things going too fast, or of commitment makes you step back to do a reality check. But the reality is you're hurting a woman who did nothing directly to create your problem. That's terribly unfair. Joe realized this when he lost Myria:

My marriage was never good. My wife was cold. A year after I left, I met Myria, who was everything my ex wasn't—loving, kind, spiritual, sexual, and independent. I was crazy about her. She wanted to take it slow but I phoned all the time. We had long talks and seeing her was unbelievable. When I signed divorce papers it hit me—I was finally on my own—maybe selling myself short getting involved so quickly. Maybe I should date more before settling down. Myria hadn't pushed for anything but she was the type I'd want to spend my life with so I panicked. I pulled back. She asked what was wrong, I said "nothing." She pushed and I pulled back more. I couldn't tell this absolutely wonderful woman who had always been straight with me that I was confused. Weeks later I forced myself to explain, but too much damage was done. She said she'd lost faith in me since I wasn't honest earlier. I hurt her badly and would do anything to have her back. I lost the chance for a relationship with the most special woman I've known.

♡ | **Connection Tip**

Rest her head on your lap (when watching TV, in bed, reading, etc.). Play with her hair, massage her temples, lightly brush her face with your fingertips.

Do you think we believe "nothing is wrong" when you build walls? We probe for answers out of fear of losing you. When we trust you emotionally and open our hearts, closing yours with nary a word crushes our faith in you, and in ourselves. How could you lead us on and then shut us out? How could we have trusted you? And the old "What's wrong with me?" sets doubts in motion. In class Vi recounted:

> When Warren began putting walls up I got scared. Normally he's loving and anxious to be with me. But he got cold one day—he wasn't there emotionally—like he wanted nothing to do with me. I assumed he didn't love me anymore. A week later he was back to loving and I was an emotional wreck. He said I'd done nothing wrong, but gave no explanation. After a few weeks of glorious loving, he got cold again. When it happens, he's like a stranger. Warren seems like two people. My friends and I referred to it as his spells. I'd have a few good weeks and then a bad one. I finally waited for a good mood and got the nerve to tell him how paranoid he made me. He was shocked that I took it personally and explained things were going badly at work and it made him feel low—not good enough for me. It was a relief. Now that we've talked about it, he doesn't do it as much.

The alienation we feel when you suddenly cool down is awful. We interpret distance as a lack of caring. We can't depersonalize your behavior enough to understand that the walls may have nothing directly to do with anything we did or your feelings for us. Am I getting through those walls a bit?

Shutting down is a defense that makes you feel safe at the moment, but it's not healthy for a relationship. Be more conscious of the damage that shutting down creates and talk to us, even if you just say something is bothering you and you need space to sort it out. Try some kindness. Not going too far away is better for you in the long run. You might be able to work through your fear instead of hiding from it.

PERSONALIZING

We personalize your actions. If you're cool, we worry you're mad at us. If we can't pinpoint why, we analyze it with friends. If you go from hot to cold, we look for what we did wrong, since we feel responsible for making a relationship work. Our fear of losing you makes us assume that we're the problem and you don't want us anymore. It builds what could be a small, impersonal thing into a major crisis. So we continuously ask what's wrong. Pam said:

> I admit I get silly worrying about Joel. I'm secure he loves me but still can't help worrying if he doesn't call when he says or if he isn't in a good mood. I wonder if I did something wrong. When I find out the real reason, I'm relieved but it doesn't stop my worrying next time. My friends do it too, and find more reasons to worry. If Joel knew the torment I put myself through each time he's not exactly as normal, he'd probably laugh at me.

We get paranoid, guys! We stress out about nothing and build it way out of proportion. Remember our insecurity? Be patient. If you care about your partner, try letting her know at least a crumb of what's making you act in ways that she reads as having a problem with her. A little reassurance is a gift of love.

PRACTICAL EMOTIONS

You keep emotions more in check than we do. John wrote, "I have emotions but still use reason to first consider the benefits and consequences of expressing them." Our emotions may have no apparent reason. We don't understand how you can be so darn reasonable with your feelings. To us, feelings spark passion, fire, movement, and expression. You may control your feelings so well that you seem like you couldn't care less. We know what we see and only understand the extent of your feelings if you let us in, at least somewhat. Julia said:

> I know men have feelings but they keep it a big secret. I hate that. My boyfriend gets angry when I accuse him of having no feelings. Yet can I read his mind? I ask questions and he gives evasive answers. I ask about his past relationships—he says they were okay and they're over. I know someone hurt him. He gets very sensitive or overreacts to certain things. I'd be more considerate if I understood, but he

won't tell. Sometimes he's warm and loving but then he gets so cold he's like a different person. That scares me.

We know you're not heartless creatures, but we often need more than you're comfortable giving. David said he has a full range of emotions but doesn't express them often. He said, "My emotions are held very close. I'm more even-keeled." Even-keeled—that indicates control. We think emotions should be exposed. We can't control ours. Controlling yours makes you seem cold.

What's the Big Deal About Keeping Feelings In? I'll Tell You!

You like fixing things, but hurt feelings aren't on your "To-Do" list. Richard explained, "The biggest problem getting through to most of us is we don't want to see our emotional problems. My friends laugh at how women work on theirs and refuse to see how bad it is to ignore them. It's taken me years to change." If you paid attention to your feelings, your achievement-oriented nature might motivate you to fix them. But you don't know how, so you ignore them.

STORED LUGGAGE

Many of you avoid references to baggage at all costs. I've asked men about unresolved problems from past relationships that affected later ones. Many of you said you had none. I'm amazed at how many guys who I knew had hang-ups said they were fine. Men who talked openly in class about situations in which they've been hurt still said they had no baggage after the class. Blinders are on tightly, even if you know the truth on another level. Jerry told me:

My last girlfriend almost destroyed me. I was so in love I let her play with me and hold sex over my head. It had started out equal. We enjoyed each other, got along well, and shared feelings. Then she started using the weaknesses I'd confessed to her against me. She played on the emotions I'd exposed during our early days. It was a painful time as I look back. She had problems and took them out on me. When we broke up it was a relief. I trusted her and now I don't

want to trust like that again. I admit that I'm totally on my guard
with women. I don't want to get close again.

Stifled feelings eventually hit you. Ignoring them increases
your capacity for anger. Yvonne said, "When men are hurt from the
past they carry scars around for life." Statistics say that today more
women are leaving men than men are leaving women. We handle
break-ups better because we have a support system. What do you
have? A dish to break? Someone to irrationally lose your temper at?
Excuses to yourself that you know don't cut it? Running away from a
woman who makes you happy? Wise up and accept that what you've
been doing isn't working well.

Women talk with friends. We vent. We cry. We get over it, at
least to a degree. You prefer to pack away feelings and forget them.
But they don't go away. You don't have to use my over-effusive gender as role models for handling emotions. Find your own way to let
them out of hiding so you can diffuse anger, resentment, hostility,
and pain. There's more than one way to deal with feelings (specific
techniques later in the chapter). Find what's comfortable, or at least
not intolerable, and work with it. If you unpack your baggage, you'll
enjoy living with a lighter load.

EMOTIONS THAT BRING YOU DOWN

When you ignore emotions, they surface in many ways. Anger is
a destructive one. It motivates you to lose your temper and pushes you
to overreact. Losing your temper is accepted in men. Jenna describes,
"In general, men keep their emotions inside until they hit a boiling
point, then explode all over their women, leaving giant piles of testosterone residue all over the room. They confuse hurt and anger. When
they feel very hurt, they express it with anger instead of admitting
vulnerability." That hurts those you care about, and you too!

As Jenna said, your response to being hurt is often anger. You
direct a lot of it at yourselves: for allowing yourself to be hurt, for letting down your guard and being vulnerable, for trusting a woman.
When you feel sad because someone hurts you, you convert it into
anger—a more manly approach. We're the opposite. When we're

angry, our feelings get hurt and we feel sad, which is considered more acceptable for women. We feel hurt by actions that make us angry. In a men's group, Edgar spoke up:

> I honestly used to think I was in good shape with emotions. I grew up in the old school of guys keeping feelings to themselves, but never saw problems until attending this group. I thought all problems in relationships were caused by women. They've let me down—I admit it hurt. But I put on my strong face and moved on. I now see that my feelings for each woman who hurt me turned into anger and I took it out on everyone. I didn't want to feel pain. I was mainly angry at myself for getting hurt—I should have known better. I'd lose my temper at a clerk if she did something that reminded me of a woman who'd hurt me. I jump on my new girlfriend's case if she does something that might remotely be done to hurt me. I'm angry at myself but I take it out on everyone. I'm trying the tools you taught us and it's working. Now I write things down and talk them out with Cindy.

Women get angry at not getting our way, when you do something negative, if we allow you to take advantage. You get angry when we criticize you, your feelings get hurt, you get dumped, you feel betrayed. Many women don't react with anger. We get hurt and tell you how we feel; we get soothed by friends; we let some of it go. You don't allow yourself to feel hurt. Those feelings often turn into anger and alienate/anger/hurt those near you who mean the most. Are you happy like this?

Taking Healthy Control of Yourself	
Don't	Do
Refuse to express what bothers you.	Talk about problems with someone you trust.
Assume negatives will just go away.	Consider therapy / a men's support group.
Think past pain won't damage now.	Become aware of how your past affects today's responses.

Jealousy is another emotion that leads to trouble. It can be unfounded and arise because you don't trust us. Women speak of boyfriends who were jealous of all men. It usually stems from insecurity, which is your problem, not ours. I had a boyfriend who was jealous of every man I talked to. He accused me of flirting with my local grocer, since I'm friendly with people I've known for years. He'd had women cheat in the past and his jealousy resulted from that. How many of you have gotten irrationally jealous? No good comes of it.

Hurt feelings come out in a variety of ways you might never expect or identify. They don't just dissipate because you want them to. Nora said, "My current beau was always with women who manipulated him and thus thinks I must always have ulterior motives for what I say." Mary offered advice after getting over her own painful relationship:

> It takes lots of patience and strength to heal emotional hurt from a relationship. Dwelling on old partners can spoil a current relationship because you're not living in the moment and not giving your best to the relationship. It's best not to get involved again for a while until you can stand on your own and be content as a single person.

If you don't trust the woman you're with, is there something concrete concerning you? If there's no reason to distrust her and you've had this experience before, identify what you're afraid of and work on it. Telling her what bothers you in a friendly, non-accusatory way (more in Chapter 6) makes you feel better in the long run. Getting cold or hostile hurts a relationship. Jenna observed, "All of our past relationships affect how we handle things in the future. The important thing is to recognize that each relationship has its own life, its own characteristics, its own positives and negatives."

HURT EMOTIONS / BAD CHOICES

Feelings affect your judgment. You may ignore how a woman hurt you but subconsciously avoid another involvement because of it. Unfortunately, it's often with women who'd make you happy. You might say, "Nah, you're crazy. Why would I avoid someone who'd make me happy?" Because women who are healthy, happy, and without a zillion problems seem dangerous if you're avoiding another broken heart. It's not funny in the long run—you often do run away. William confessed in a class:

> I've been hurt a few times and swore it wouldn't happen again. I recognize what you've talked about as something I've been doing recently—avoiding women I could fall hard for. I admit I don't want to go through a broken heart again. I was seeing someone recently— a terrific gal. Sheryl has a good career, nice friends, and a great attitude. She had no bad qualities I could see. She respected my feelings and didn't make demands. So what did I do? I slept with a woman who comes to me when she needs help. I told Sheryl about it. Let it slip out, probably subconsciously to push her back a bit, but she stopped seeing me. Said I'm dangerous if I sleep with women like that. She's right. The other woman is a mess and sleeps around. I feel like I self-destructed a potential relationship for sex with a woman who's messed up. Now I'm seeing the messed up one. I can't stop myself.

A bitch or a woman with problems may seem safer than a healthy one. You probably won't get too involved and you have an excuse for a fast exit. If you've been hurt, you may bond with an emotionally bruised woman. But it won't make you happy. Alex said men have totally unrealistic expectations, especially after being hurt. "Men have this idea. You see it in movies—a man is saving a woman. We feel if we save one ourselves then she won't leave us. Wrong! That's fiction." Bonding on negatives doesn't lead to a positive relationship. You can get some of your needs met in an unhealthy relationship. You feel needed, have a project to fix, and satisfy your sexual appetite. A healthy relationship is more satisfying in the long run.

Women Who Play Therapist

As stereotypical nurturers, we love finding ways to "help" you. We pick your brains and offer a sympathetic ear to get you to open up. Larry asked a question that I've heard a zillion varieties of—"Why do women encourage us to spill our guts to them?" It's not your imagination that we analyze you and offer solutions. Since we believe we're better at handling emotional issues, many of us can't resist playing therapist. But playing therapist can be a form of manipulation with "good intentions."

THE SECURITY OF THERAPY

We encourage you to open up, hoping it'll bring us closer. We like giving you support. Sharing feelings and experiences infers trust—we want you to trust us. Then, with the help of friends (co-analysts), we analyze the value of your trust in relation to what we assume your feelings for us must be. Carrie told a class:

> I was so happy when Jeremy shared a lot of personal things on our fifth date. He seemed so trusting. My friends agreed it was a good sign. They pushed me to get him to open up even more. I encouraged him—supported and nurtured him—made suggestions about how he could handle different feelings. I felt so close to him at first that I settled in for a long-term relationship. Then he started cooling down. It made no sense but eventually he jumped down my throat about my analyzing him. It's over now. So much for trust.

A problem with our getting you to open up is that when it happens, trust may be given prematurely. If you've spent most of your life not sharing feelings, a kind, sympathetic ear can be a source of solace at the moment. But, you may stop in your tracks after realizing you've opened up to a woman you don't know well enough to trust, no matter how nice she seems. Many of you bolt at that point, leaving your therapist and her friends trying to analyze what went wrong.

Women often play therapist for the wrong reasons. We want to increase our security, thinking if we earn your confidence we'll be closer; if you become dependent on our support, you'll need us. Some of us have a misguided view that if we let you dump problems on us, you won't leave. You know the deal on that.

SPILLING YOUR GUTS

We'd love you to spill your guts, thinking it develops trust when you share personal feelings and experiences. We don't understand it's better to take our time. We sometimes play therapist because we think we can make you a better man. The trouble for you is that it's OUR version of better. Gary told me:

> *Harriet started asking questions subtly. It felt good to talk about my old girlfriend. I had a lot of anger. The more I talked, the more she asked. Later I was uncomfortable with how much she knew. I stopped talking and she bugged me more. I kept thinking about what she knew and felt I didn't know her well enough. I broke up with her. Now I'm seeing Susan. I started off not saying anything. Then I told her a little as you recommended. I asked her to respect my limits and she did. I'm starting to trust Susan and am telling her more. I feel good about telling her stuff when I'm ready, not because she pushes.*

My recommendation: Don't open up too quickly, even if she seems special. It may feel good to talk things over. But it can damage a relationship if a solid foundation of trust isn't there yet, or if you share things you may regret. Don't talk about your exes at the beginning, unless it's positive. Communicating past history and emotional baggage is one instance where communication should be limited. Share slowly, no matter how much she encourages you to open up. Let a little bit out each time. Use compliments as a diversion!

Controlling Your Need to Control

A common complaint from women is that many of you can be very controlling. Your need to control a relationship may be tied to stereotypes of men needing to take charge or take care of us. It develops from your program to be responsible for our welfare. When things aren't as *you* think they should be, you try to "correct" the situation. Your program is to provide and protect but some of you go overboard. Control may seem the best way to live up to the traditional male role in a relationship, but it creates tension and is unfair to your partner.

 Connection Tip

Put on some soft music and ask her to dance.

THE NEED TO CONTROL

Both sexes like having control over people in their lives. You do it more since we tolerate more, at least at first, when we want you in our lives. We let you take charge and bitch to friends about it. You won't tolerate a controlling woman as readily. It's bad for either sex.

Insecurity motivates you to control what you can. If you're losing control over parts of your life, especially your job, controlling us can make you feel better. You may put us down to keep us insecure and manipulated, and our low self-esteem keeps us there. Do you resent your partner if she has a better job, a boss who thinks the world of her when yours doesn't, an easier schedule, supportive friends, etc.? To feel control over something, you may dictate what goes on in your personal life, with no regard for us. Alfred reported in a group:

> Women before Mary called me a control freak. I was being a man. My dad was in charge at home—now it was my responsibility. I work hard for no appreciation and felt I should make decisions at home. I recently married Mary. She got angry when I made decisions in her best interests. I insisted we do certain activities on the weekend, and saw it as nice for her. She called it coercion. I got Chinese food I thought we'd enjoy together last week and she refused to eat it. Said I should have asked what she'd like. I heard men in the group talk about being controlling and how they weren't happy in the long run. I asked Mary what she wanted and listened for the first time. She said a partnership, not a dictatorship. Her father controlled and she'd watch her mother be miserable. She had no intention of going through that. If I needed to control someone, it wouldn't be her. It's been hard but I've asked her to let me know when I'm controlling. I'm trying to stop.

CONTROLLING FEARS

Fear motivates us to control whatever we can. If someone hurt you in your past (and who hasn't?), you may be more cautious with everyone else you're involved with. Many people try controlling as much as possible to avoid getting hurt again.

I had a boyfriend who was likable but always wanted his way. Past girlfriends had let him down—he wouldn't let it happen again. He had one way of doing things—HIS. All other ways were wrong. Some of his controlling was under the guise of caring, or given with such enthusiasm it was hard to say "no." Eventually my resentment grew. I tried to talk about respecting my needs and feelings but he closed up. I had to let go of an otherwise good man because he wouldn't stop expecting everything his way.

I had lunch with a friend and told her about him. She said, "He's doing what I've been in therapy for years to work on and I'm still working on it." She asked about his childhood—it was similar to hers. They'd both had many rules and little warmth. Each saw their parent of the opposite sex as in charge. My friend explained:

> *Many things were out of my control growing up and I always felt scared. As I got older, I believed if I compacted my life I could handle it better. For years I created a box around it, believing if I controlled everything I'd feel safe. My world was insulated. I had one way of thinking. People close to me had to do things my way or they couldn't fit into the box. My life was a nice neat package. Nothing was allowed in that didn't fit my mold. Your boyfriend is doing the same. He's scared and wants to mold you into a woman who'll fit into his box of security. Years of therapy taught me to focus on control over myself only. I take risks and enjoy life much more. I still try to control my boyfriend too much but he knows I'm trying so he's patient with me. Letting myself out of the box was hard.*

Do you see yourself putting a box around your world? Do you expect your partner to do things your way? If you've been accused of being too controlling, lighten up for your own sake. Write down your fears (more on this later in the chapter). Putting worries on paper helps put them in perspective. Read them objectively and understand that each can be dealt with. If fear motivates us to be controlling, then we're not really in control. The fear is. You may feel safer putting your life in nice, tidy order but it's not healthy or fair to others. It's not fun either. If you face your fears they do go away!

AGENDA FOR TWO

It's okay to be strong, independent, and decisive if you're flexible enough to remember there's two people in a relationship. You can't make all decisions. Just as I tell women not to play mother, don't play father. A healthy relationship is a partnership. When you tell your partner what you think, ask what she thinks before making your decision a done deal. Practice compromising. There are many ways to do things. Your way is only one of them.

Some of you make decisions based on what seems logical. If you believe your way is good for us, you may not discuss it. You make plans without consulting us. Women complain about guys who assume their decisions for both are fine. That's disrespectful to your partner. It tells her you don't value her opinions. Jordan almost lost his girlfriend when he ignored her input:

> *May agreed to move in with me. My life got hectic a month before moving day. I didn't have much free time. May complained I made no time for her. I kept thinking that once we lived together it would all sort itself out. I was so convinced that I ignored her requests for more phone calls and quality time together. I did what I felt needed to be done and was thrown when she left a message that she wasn't moving in. She'd have talked to me about it in person but I gave her no opportunity. After I promised to make decisions with her, not for her, she agreed to stay with me. Control isn't worth losing May over.*

Be responsible for you. Healthy people only control themselves. No matter how much you love her, no matter how much she seems to need help, no matter how much you believe your way is right, being controlling causes resentment in the long run. She's responsible for herself. Offer advice IF she's receptive. But you have no right to insist, demand, or implement changes that she isn't open to. It can push her away. There's a big difference between controlling everything in your life and being in control of you. The latter is the only control you should strive for. If she doesn't want everything your way, backing off is the best direction. Then ask what she thinks.

Many of you stoically endure all problems by controlling/ manipulating until you alienate us. Talk about why you may have tried to control things and what you feel responsible for. Let us give you support. When your lady gets fed up with your controlling, you may allow alcohol, drugs, depression, etc. to control you. Is it worth it? You know the answer.

Getting in Touch with Emotions in a Comfortable Way

It's not necessary to emulate women to get more in touch with your feelings. You're taught to be in control, but emotions need sorting out. Punching a wall won't make you feel nearly as good as telling us why you feel a certain way and letting it go. Most of us would accept less emotional expression than you think. Find your own comfortable way to express feelings. Sharing some thoughts will bring you closer. She doesn't have to know everything. You can still own your feelings.

Fear of showing emotions in front of us isn't unfounded. It's still hard for some of us to accept too much emotion in a guy, no matter how much we say we want it. We're just not used to it. But there's a balance between not being in touch with your feelings at all and going overboard—find your comfort zone. We need to see more sensitivity in men; it shows that you're human, and your heart isn't cold or shut down. Making the effort to give us some of what we ask for won't drain you. It makes us much happier and also makes you happier—not holding everything in feels.

Do you want true intimacy with your partner? That means letting her in, at least a little—sharing what you feel, your dreams, your goals, and eventually your fears. Intimacy builds trust. I encourage you to take your time about letting her get to know you on the inside. Take baby steps—impart small bits at a time. If you slowly build intimacy, your connection to her will grow stronger and sweeter.

FOURTEEN STEPS TO EMOTIONAL WELL-BEING

The following are steps you can take to get in touch with yourself. Some are baby steps that can lead to grown-up rewards. Some may feel like heavy steps over fire. Take your time. Put at least your toe forward to get started. It will put you on a path to a more open relationship with your partner, and more importantly, with yourself.

1. *Acknowledge that you have more feelings than you allow to surface.* Admitting you have feelings takes courage if you've spent a lifetime stifling them. It's a risk to show vulnerability. We know you're scared of getting hurt, losing control, not looking manly, etc., if you let feelings out of the bag. That's being human. Don't do more than you can handle at one time but do something!

2. *Redefine the macho outlook.* It takes a real man to face feelings. Behind tough facades are insecure men. Do you think that macho and courage are synonymous? Think again. It takes strength to shed the protection of a macho front and find solutions to emotional problems.

3. *Trace back where your attitude about emotional issues comes from.* Figuring out why you can't deal with emotional stuff provides a better chance of getting past it. Is it a program from childhood? Were you teased for crying? Do friends reinforce the stereotype that men should ignore emotions? Remind yourself that you can respond differently, with the power to control your actions and reactions.

4. *Accept that it's okay to be vulnerable.* You don't have to always be strong. Relax sometimes and take off your armor. Carrying the burden of your emotions is exhausting. I'm not encouraging you to give your trust easily or to everyone. But you can start slowly. Test the waters and baby-step your way to opening up with at least one special person. Try it on before you wear it regularly. You may be reluctant to open up too much, and that's okay. Pick and choose situations with people you trust and allow yourself to be human!

5. *Stop living in the past.* When we let old baggage affect what we do today, we're living in the past (more to follow). Slowly unpacking old suitcases helps heal old wounds so you can interact with your present partner on the basis of what you feel now. Staying closed makes it hard to have a healthy, fully satisfying relationship.

♡ | *Connection Tip*

Invite her to play hooky from work. Go to a movie, go bowling, have a picnic, or take a walk. Hold hands and enjoy doing things while others work. Make love in the afternoon.

6. *Don't punish new women for old hurts.* If you let what someone did to you in the past affect the present, your current partner suffers the repercussions. That's unfair! When fear of getting hurt again drives you, reactions to us are based on defenses developed with women before us. That hurts. It also hurts you because you may push aside or hurt a woman who could be a loving partner. I've experienced guys pulling back suddenly, getting cool, and getting an attitude, usually when things were heating up or feeling great. I don't like paying the price for what someone else did to hurt you! None of us do. Sheila elaborated:

> *I've actually had to scream at a boyfriend that I'm not his last girl-friend and to stop punishing me for what someone else did. My friends have stories of men who suddenly got snotty or cold because of a harmless comment or action that reminded them of someone who hurt them. That's not fair! My current boyfriend is highly sensitive because of past women and I'm tired of getting crap for what THEY did. Men need to get over it and respond objectively to what's going on in OUR relationship, not those from the past!*

Become aware of where your emotional response to things your current partner says or does comes from. Did what she say remind you of a past love? Did your fear of being hurt again cause you to over-react? Remind yourself that she didn't do what the one who hurt you did. Stop yourself from letting it hurt your present relationship by going slow and letting her earn your trust slowly. But keep reminding yourself that she isn't the other woman.

7. *Learn from what hurt you in the past.* Think about painful incidents in the past without blaming yourself. What may have caused them to happen? How did you become so vulnerable? Did you jump in too fast? In that case, be careful and go slower next time. Did you tell her too much about you? Open up in increments with your next girlfriend. Did she cheat on you? Why do you think she may have cheated? Were you neglecting her? You can keep that from happening. Identifying what behavior led to a disappointment or heartbreak in the past gives you a chance to do things differently today. George recognized this:

> I was in a bad relationship five years ago. Bridget played with me before ending it. I was hung up on her and gave her what she wanted. We went fast—I didn't stop for air or pay attention to details. When we broke up I was nervous but jumped in with Carin. It also got intense fast and later I saw things I should have seen earlier. After Carin I'd had enough. Two relationships had ended painfully. I dated casually and hurt a few women who were nice by sabotaging any chance of something good happening to avoid getting hurt. When I met Claire, I didn't want to lose her. I thought about what had screwed up my other relationships—going too fast and not getting to know her along the way. So I went very slow with Claire but didn't sabotage our chance as I'd done before. We might get married. I need more time but I'm less scared.

8. Set new boundaries. Allow more breathing room for your feelings. Practice with female friends. We won't judge you as much as other guys might. Don't let your partner push you too fast when you give her a little. If she complains when you make an effort, ask for patience. We can be demanding—give us a little and we often want more. Remind her *nicely* that you're trying. Do it at your own pace, but do it! Open up slowly to develop trust. Find your way as you go.

9. Find your own comfort level. There's a big difference between depending on a woman and sharing a life with her. Absorb this distinction! Feeling dependent on someone goes against your program to be in charge. You may worry that if she's privy to your feelings you may lose power in the relationship. I won't say it can't happen because it can. But by trusting her a little at a time, you can test your level of comfort. Sharing feelings isn't all or nothing. Share a little. See how it feels. Share a bit more. Clark agreed:

Once we moved in together, Shawna complained I never told her what I was feeling. I was let down by my last few ladies and thought I knew better. I acted the macho role and refused personal questions. I joined this group because Shawna was ready to leave me. She called me a cold stranger. I was at a loss. I avoided emotions to keep from getting hurt but was losing the lady I loved. You made me realize I was hurting more from not speaking to Shawna about my past. I finally talked a little and asked her to be patient. When she saw I was trying, she eased up some. Telling my lovely lady about how I'd been hurt was a huge relief. I still haven't told her everything. She's happier and I feel much better. I learned when a woman earns your trust as Shawna did, it's cool to open up.

10. **Be clear about what you need.** If we ask, "What's wrong?" and you need space to think something through, say so. When things are going well, explain that you like sorting out things alone and can't talk until you're ready, this is how you prefer to handle problems, and it has nothing to do with her. Ask to have this need respected. Tell her how much it would mean if she doesn't take it personally.

11. **Give her at least an idea of what's going on when you have something on your mind that's affecting you.** Since many emotional responses are triggered by our not understanding how you feel, an effort to clue us in is reassuring. We get scared that you have a problem with us and feel reassured knowing it's something else. We can't read minds, although we try to by second-guessing and analyzing. Understanding you more allows her to feel secure. Explain what's going on inside of you (even if it's just gas!) to help her relax. You may get peace in exchange for an honest discussion.

12. **Explain so she understands.** You and your partner can get into the habit of thinking about where your needs come from. When you share the feelings behind what you need, it helps make sense of what you want, which makes them easier to accept. Explaining motives for something you want or being specific about why a situation bothers you may motivate her to make an effort to give you more of what you ask for. Barney gave a good example of this in a support group:

I used to tell Evelyn that when I came home from work, I wanted dinner ready and her undivided attention so I could tell her about my day. I'd insist as the man of the house who worked hard all day, I should get my way. She worked too but her job seemed easy compared to mine. She rarely gave me what I wanted without an attitude and coming home was unpleasant for both of us. After being in the group, I realized that dinner and my wife's attention were important because of my childhood. My father worked two jobs but always came home for dinner. It was his way of letting the family know how much we meant to him. We always shared stories about our day. It was a special time for me and I wanted that with Evelyn. When I acknowledged that she worked hard too and explained what dinner meant to me, she gave me a big hug and I've been having my dinners ever since.

If Barney hadn't explained to Evelyn, he'd still have a grouchy wife and cold potatoes. Now she knows he wasn't trying to be difficult. Barney never thought about why he needed his routine so Evelyn saw him as unreasonable. Now she's happy to please him. Why do things that we bristle over when understanding makes us more reasonable. Encourage her to clarify why specific things are important to her. It establishes cooperation that can last a lifetime.

13. *Remember that all women are jerks until proven otherwise too!* Open up a little. I tell women that all men are jerks until proven otherwise. All women are jerks until proven otherwise too. That expression means don't trust someone until they've earned it. Don't fall for the initial impression someone gives when they may be on their best behavior. That's how we set ourselves up to be hurt. Let them prove otherwise with actions over time. It means go slowly, but go! We shouldn't give trust away easily in any circumstance. It needs to be earned. But it can't be earned if we don't take risks.

14. *Learn to forgive.* Forgiveness is critical in a relationship (more to follow). Grudges stimulate anger. Talk out what bothers you and move on. If we admit to being wrong and try to make up for it, forgive an occasional goof and don't take it personally. But don't accept constant unfair behavior. In that case, stop getting angry and think about ending the relationship. You shouldn't be with someone who hurts you regularly. But if you trust her and don't think she's purposely hurting you, forgive and let it go.

 Romantic Tip

> Make a list of the nonsexual details about her that you like—her smile; sense of humor; how she hugs; her cheerfulness, intelligence, kindness to others; her serious look when she's working. Let her see it—make her day!

LIVING IN THE PRESENT

I learned a great lesson from Dr. Peter Reznik, a doctor of health psychology in New York City. He taught me that if actions are based on past experiences, you hold onto the fears and limitations of the person you were then. My success increased after putting the past in perspective. I'm a stronger woman. I've used this technique many times, especially with guys. Reminding myself I'm a different woman than in past relationships keeps past fears from affecting my present ones too much. Each woman you're with is different from past ones. Remind yourself that you're more enlightened and can handle yourself better.

Dr. Reznik explained that we're an accumulation of our experiences. An important tool for handling problems is to deal with what *is*, not what *was*. Learn why past experiences happened and prevent them from recurring in a healthier way than by avoiding intimacy. Lots of stuff happened since then. Your life isn't the same. You're not either. Understand why it happened so you can approach women differently—not just avoid closeness. Emotional memories don't have to haunt you. Live for now—give your current lady an unbiased shot. Imagine a happier scenario because you've found the cause of past problems, learned from them, and left them in the past.

OPEN YOUR FEELINGS

I want to share a tool that's great for sorting out feelings—writing. Using a pen to sort feelings can be incredibly therapeutic, and easy! Forget hating to write for school. This kind of writing can be a private weapon for keeping healthy control over your emotions. Writing feelings down is a great relief. It gets things off your chest. And, no one has to see it.

I've given clients writing assignments and they've been skeptical—until they tried it. When we have anger, disappointment, guilt, fear, and other emotions, we often keep them close to the surface to protect ourselves. Sometimes we think about troubling issues so we don't forget and repeat mistakes. Bad emotions can cause physical ailments—stomachaches—acid indigestion—ulcers—headaches. Putting feelings on paper takes the pressure off and allows us to put them into perspective. We can look at them. We don't have to hold on to them inside because they're recorded if we need a reminder. Often once we write them down, they become less important. Elliot tried it and reported:

> I didn't know why I'd always snap at Liv but I couldn't control it. One thing wrong and I'd lose it. It's happened in all my relationships. Things that had bothered me about each woman I'd been involved with built up when each relationship ended. You suggested I make three lists—things about my mother that made me angry, things about women that made me angry, and things I like about Liv. I was surprised at the long list about my mother. I realized how many things angered me as a child, and it continues. I didn't understand why you had me write about her until I wrote about other women— many things I got angry about reminded me of what my mother did. What a revelation. After a week of adding to the lists, I read them over and discovered that most of the things women did to make me angry didn't seem as important now as they did. I'd been looking for trouble with Liv. She's a good woman. The list about her put that in focus. It was like magic—once I wrote everything down and studied the lists, I was consciously less angry. My stomach problems are much better. It was like I took the anger out of myself and stored it on paper. That's how you described it and that's how it felt. I plan to do more writing exercises.

You download documents to discs or CDs to make room on your computer's hard drive. Writing things down cleans out your own. Lists help us see things more clearly and get things off our chests. I don't sleep well if something is on my mind. Now I bring a pad and pen to bed to write down whatever is bothering me. I've written letters to guys I was angry with, saying how I felt, but never sent them. Saving my feelings on paper helps me sleep. After writing, I don't feel so angry. I recommend writing individual lists of things that scare you or make you feel angry, guilty, jealous, worried, etc. Try one (or all). Keep each topic separate. Write what you feel about something, or write as if you were speaking to a person. It's your call. Read them later and learn about your feelings. Getting your anger down on paper can get it out of your heart. At times I've burned the letters and my anger went up in smoke! Peter said during a session, "I made a list of everything that made me angry and one about my fears. Wow, they were long. But once I read them over I felt I could deal with them. Thank you."

If you get angry at your partner, write everything down before confrontations. Walk away for a short time to cool down and spell out on paper what made you angry before speaking about it. Writing it down can diffuse your anger and put it more into perspective. It gives you a chance to think about what to say in a way she may understand, which is most important. Then tell her why you're angry. Try this with friends and colleagues too.

Practicing Forgiveness

Practicing forgiveness is resolving anger and moving on. If you don't forgive, anger can lead to resentment that damages relationships. If she does something that bothers you, see if her response is acceptable and forgive. You put women down for apologizing a lot. Although we can take it to an extreme, saying "I'm sorry" makes us all feel better. Forgiveness is synonymous with trust. If you trust her word and believe she's sincerely sorry, forgive her. Carl said:

Before Darlene, I was nailed by several girlfriends who betrayed me. I began trusting less. It got hard accepting apologies for nasty things. When I met Darlene I waited for her to hurt me. When she canceled a date at the last minute with a good excuse, my anger stayed for days. I gave her a hard time. Then she forgot to tell me she was working late. When I finally got her, I was furious. She apologized and I ranted. She said I must have had bad experiences if I couldn't allow myself to trust her enough to forgive her mistakes. She reminded me she'd never given a reason to doubt her and if I wanted to punish someone for what others did, I could leave. She was right. I apologized and she forgave me for being a jerk. That taught me how important it is to forgive. I almost lost a great gal.

In your need to always be right, it's hard to admit you're wrong. Acknowledging a mistake or unfair accusation will score high with your partner. You're known for not being able to say "I'm sorry." Many of you have to force an apology, even if you know that you're wrong. So force it! It's harder to forgive a guy who won't sincerely say he's sorry. Even if you don't believe you did anything wrong or purposely hurt her, say you're sorry it hurt her. When a guy hurts me and spends all his energy defending what he did without showing compassion for my feelings, it's hard to let go of bad ones. Forgiveness allows us to leave anger behind. Once you see how much good it does, you'll appreciate being able to forgive someone you care about and be forgiven.

More Tips for Healthy Emotions

Consciously appreciate the good things about your partner by writing them down. Does she get on your nerves? Why are you with her? Focus on the positives. Think about how nice it is to see her.

Do you come home stressed, thinking about what your boss did or how much work you have? Change that! Don't bring problems home and take them out on your partner. Calm yourself first. Write down what bothers you. When you leave a stressful situation, get in the habit of doing slow breathing and listening to relaxing music on your iPod or CD player. Taking problems out on us serves no constructive purpose. Talking them out might. Leaving them behind for a relaxing evening definitely does.

Be open-minded about her complaints. Several times I've gotten a response I call the *Popeye Syndrome*—"I am what I am"—from a guy who'd done me wrong. Yes, we should accept you for who you are but that doesn't make all your actions fair. When we tell you about something that bothers us, get in the habit of listening objectively. Actually thinking about what's said instead of getting defensive can make you more accepting. A little compassion will get you far. Ignoring us gets you grief.

 Sharing Exercise

Give her ten *uninterrupted* minutes to talk about whatever she needs to. Make an effort to listen carefully. Then you take ten minutes to share what you need without interruption. After, discuss what was shared.

I want to share a technique I always recommend for couples. Ask to sit down with her one night each week in a relaxed setting. Set a nice mood, perhaps with wine or tea and candles. Share your feelings in a peaceful way. Clearing the air doesn't have to be an unpleasant or confrontational experience. You can share in different ways. Take turns explaining how you feel about things. Each of you can write your feelings down in advance. Either exchange your lists or read them to each other. Then nicely discuss what you've learned.

Getting more in touch with emotions doesn't have to be a disruptive change in your program. Find your comfort zone. Accept that having bad experiences is inevitable when dealing with the opposite sex. Relationships always have snags. But you can fix or patch problems and put them behind you with the right tools. I hope you'll give it a shot. You'll be more in control of yourself if you do.

6

COMMUNICATION BREAKDOWN:
FINDING A COMMON LANGUAGE

Your partner says those four words you dread, "We need to talk." You look for ways to bolt because you hate this. She begins explaining what's bothering her and your defenses rise. You try to respond as well as you can but she wants more. You get angrier but make the effort to say what you think she wants. She complains you're lousy at communicating. You don't get it. Don't you communicate well with your friends? Why doesn't she appreciate the effort you're making? In the past, you never tried at all. Now that you are, it's not enough. You wonder why women accuse you of not communicating when you are. It's not fair. Why doesn't she understand that I am communicating? What does she want? ～

A key to a successful relationship is good communication. Yet communication problems are a big complaint from both sexes. We complain that you don't communicate. You get angry because you are communicating—it's just not how she wants it. The concept of communication gets muddied as we interpret it one way and you interpret it another.

What's good communication? It's interaction where one is speaking while the other listens, and vice versa. Good communication isn't throwing words or humoring us by pretending to listen when you're not. Some of you are pros at that! Good communication is paying real attention to what the other person says and having a thoughtful response. That can be hard for both sexes. Women often don't shut up long enough to listen and you often don't want to listen because you don't like what we're saying! Let's change!

Different Dialects

Women don't always understand that communication doesn't mean doing it *our* way. You may think it's okay to ignore us, while nodding to simulate paying attention. Are you paying attention now? You should if you want one of the keys to pleasing us. Real communication isn't painful when you learn the art and modify it so it feels comfortable. According to Jenna, good communication is "when a man speaks and listens equally; when he pays attention completely; when he brings up something you said off-hand from days/weeks ago—that tells you he was really listening. When it doesn't feel like pulling teeth."

COMMUNICATION NEEDS

In general, each sex has a different style of expressing thoughts. You say less to get a point across, using a minimum of words. We embellish and can go into more detail than you deem necessary. Details enhance our conversations. Neither sex is right or wrong. We like using (and sometimes overusing) words. You have less need to verbally express feelings. Getting carried away by emotions motivates our giving verbal dissertations. You complain that once we get started it can be hard to stop us. Many of you ask why we like talking so much. It gives us a chance to sort our thoughts by hearing them out loud. Feedback from you helps. It's not hard to give us at least some of what we want. Alex has his own philosophy:

> A woman's need for communication can be placated by simply saying something. Often it doesn't matter what. If it's apologetic, all the better. I see men saying what women want to hear all the time and don't mean it—they just go through the motions. It turns my stomach how easily they can get over on women and the women accept what they give.

I'd rather you do it in a sincere way. Lip service isn't honest. Our needs aren't hard to meet. Here's the deal. We like to talk about more personal stuff. Many of you don't. We won't always have a point when we say something. That's your thing. Since talking enhances the intimacy we crave, we engage you in conversations that seem to go nowhere in your practical mind. We see conversations bringing us closer together, so they're important to us. Humor us a little. We enjoy talking to you for the sake of connecting with you through words. Personal conversations deepen the friendship between you and your partner. While chatting about other people, their feelings and their situations may seem trivial to you, it feels intimate to share with you.

COMMUNICATION STYLES

Men and women communicate differently with their own sex. Women have long, intimate conversations with each other. Yours may be more casual and much shorter. Lee said, "Men are more literal. Women are working communications on more levels." We make eye contact, especially since we face each other when we speak to other women. Often men speak sitting next to each other with no eye contact, in a bar, at a ball game, or in a conference room.

Be Careful What You Say!		
WHAT YOU SAY	WHAT YOU MEAN	WHAT SHE HEARS
"I'll talk to you later."	You'll talk to her some time in the future.	You'll talk to her later today.
"I need to clean the garage."	You'll clean the garage some day.	You'll clean the garage ASAP.
"Should we skip dessert?"	You're too full from the entrée.	She is too fat for dessert.

You complain we hassle you if you speak in the same manner as you do to other guys. Your style can be coarser than ours. We may find some of your language offensive. Your friends would agree that it's part of being a guy. Ours would say you should speak to us nicely. A middle ground can be reached to establish fair boundaries, such as no foul language and no yelling. Barry found a compromise:

> *Maggie criticized how I spoke after we moved in together, saying I was bringing home bad habits from the guys. I curse with friends and did it with her. She got angry and called me disrespectful. I was okay being on good behavior when we were just dating. But when we lived together—hey, that was my home and I wanted to be comfortable. I resented Maggie picking on how I spoke and probably did it more for spite. We went to a family party a few months ago. I was with Maggie and my mom in the kitchen and my uncle started talking to me the way I speak to my friends—loud, with foul language. Mom jumped in and said there were ladies present. Uncle Tom laughed but I got upset about him speaking that way with my mom. Maggie just looked at me and I got it! Now I'm more careful—I can't help myself sometimes but she's okay if she knows I'm trying.*

Getting Your Point Across Without an Argument

You can communicate effectively, even with us. It's worth the effort when you get a response you like! I've put together my own Ten Commandments of Good Communication, modifying the ones I give women to suit your style of communication. Some may seem obvious, annoying, silly, or plain dumb. But they work, so give them a chance. Following my commandments can enable you to maintain effective communication on the most objective level possible, without too much effort. Isn't that a great combination?

Ten Commandments of Good Communication for Men

1. Find a peaceful time to talk. If possible, avoid serious talk when you're annoyed, rushed, or distracted. If it means waiting a day or two to calm down, have more time, or focus on what to say, wait to get your point across under the best of conditions. But, don't use this as an excuse to postpone talking indefinitely. The most conducive time for objective listening is when you're both in a good mood. If this isn't possible, go for the best mood under the circumstances. Postponing discussion for too long leads to more problems. Be a man and find the right time.

2. *Stick to the point and say enough to clearly make your point.* When you make an effort to open up to your partner, choose your battles carefully. It's easy to get carried away when you're finally in the groove of communicating. Don't bring up all the annoying issues you've kept to yourself until then. It's tempting to include it all so you won't have to communicate again for a LONG time. Don't. Say what you really mean. We see you as speaking a different language. Nora said, "Sometimes men are indirect—they say things like 'Well if I *was* angry about that then I *would* . . .' Say you're angry!" Don't use generic words to avoid spelling out what you think. An ex-boyfriend used the word "fun" to describe all his feelings. It threw me at first. Instead of saying "I care" he'd say I was fun. Sex was fun. My cooking him dinner was fun. Eventually I accepted "fun" was complimentary. Get a thesaurus if words don't come! Use as few words as possible, but make your point clearly. We tend to say too much—communication overkill. You, on the other hand, may throw a few words out without clarification and call it a night. We HATE being left hanging! Ian advises, "Be direct, clear, and ask more questions. Tell her exactly what you want with examples to clarify." Be specific about what you want us to know and clear when you respond to us. We're used to details so give us at least a few. If we ask for clarification, suck in your breath and try again. Patience!

3. Speak with the same respect that you'd want for yourself. Think about how you'd feel if the tone and attitude you're using were used on you. Is it respectful or condescending? Listen to yourself. How would you feel if someone spoke to you that way? Becoming aware of how we communicate enables us to do it more effectively. Pay more attention to yourself. You may hear things in your tone you won't like and may not have been aware of. I got rid of the naggy, whiny tone used for speaking to men after I consciously heard myself

speak with it for the first time. You may not like what you hear when you listen to yourself. I didn't and it motivated me to find other ways of getting my point across.

4.   Start and end with a positive statement. Since we bristle when you tell us something you mean as constructive, set a positive tone first. Getting defensive during a serious talk affects how we hear it. When I know someone is going to say something that I may not like, my mind formulates a defense instead of listening objectively. Help your partner stay open by saying something nice first, such as "I'm happy that we're together" or "I'm glad I can share things with you." Her guard will more likely go down. You know what we like to hear. When you're done, woo her into a positive mindset for considering what you said with something sweet or complimentary. "You're great to talk to" is a good one. Segue into issues you want to bring up after bringing her guard down. Don't lie or manipulate her with words. Sincerely find something you mean and say it. Then end on a positive note to help her absorb the message more objectively. Leave her with a good feeling. That makes you feel good too.

5. *Explain, don't complain.* Criticism is an intimacy buster. I said earlier that we don't appreciate constructive criticism. If you want her to listen with an open mind, don't lecture, blame, criticize, or talk down to her. Explain by just stating the facts. Don't get too personal. If she thinks you're telling her what to do she may get put off. Communicate in a way that she feels she has choices.

6. *Use positive words instead of negatives to say the same thing.* Soften the blow, guys! A friendlier/nicer/more positive vehicle can make what you have to say easier to swallow. For example, instead of saying "You're doing that wrong," say "May I suggest another way?" Choosing less negative words allows a better shot of getting her to see your point of view. "I don't like" can be "I'd prefer."

7. *Ask her to consider your point of view instead of telling her to do it your way.* We won't change because you say you know better. Ask to have your suggestions considered. Our antennae go up if we

suspect you're trying to control us. Respecting her right to be herself and make her own decisions can keep her mind more open. Neither sex should expect the other to change because they want their way. But if things bother you, ask her to be more aware of how she makes you feel. "Please work with me, honey" is better than snapping at her. Tell her specifically why something annoys you. For example, if she attacks you with complaints as you walk in from work, state why it bothers you, without an attitude. Explain how burnt you are—if she waits until you're settled, you'll listen with less irritation. But don't expect total compliance. Ask how she'd like to be reminded if she forgets, instead of barking at her to shut up. A phrase like "Remember I need to unwind first" or a kiss followed by "I love you" and a quick exit from the room can push her pause button. If she waits, thank her for being patient. Asking for more awareness about specific things you have a problem with instead of demanding change will get you more of what you need.

8. Be patient. Don't expect a good response because you finally communicated. She may want time to think. She'll probably still say more than you'd like and prod for too many details. Patiently listening for a few minutes can placate her need to share. Force yourself to answer at least some questions. Patience really is a virtue, one that can please your woman in ways that you'll ultimately be pleased too!

9. Pay attention to what she says. We often forget that communication includes listening, which is considered a skill (more to follow). You're not known for being skillful at it, but you can learn! Many of you said the best way to placate a woman is to agree with everything she says or say what she wants to hear. That averts problems in the short run but she'll eventually know you didn't mean it. It's hard for some of you to sincerely acknowledge all of a chatty woman's comments and questions. But get out of the habit of "yessing" us. Jennifer told me, "Hector wasn't paying attention at all. I was trying to save my marriage and he was agreeing without hearing. He agreed when I said I was moving out. Now he's trying to get my attention to come back—it's too late." We talk a lot but aren't a bunch of ditzes. We know what you're doing but don't know how to change

it—except walk out on you. Take her more seriously if you value her being in your life.

10. *Respond to what she says.* If she tells you something, answer her. We need feedback. Grunts and body movements don't cut it. An ambiguous word or two doesn't either. Amy said good communication is "coming out of a conversation or argument with a mutual understanding of what went on . . . not feeling like you're banging your head into a wall, or that one of you is speaking a foreign language." Make an effort, even if we don't seem satisfied. Assure her that you're trying. Amy explained, "The biggest frustration I have is hearing words come out of their mouths . . . 'I'll call you later—tomorrow—Monday; I'll do x, y, z; I'll be there at ___' and seeing absolutely ZERO follow-through. I'm real big on consideration and if a guy's words don't match his actions, then I don't even want him to open his mouth." If you give communication a shot and she's grumbling, tell her you'll keep trying if she's patient. It's the best you can do for now.

♡ | **Connection Tip**

Before you speak to her about something that bothers you, ask yourself if you'd talk to your best friend the way you're about to do with your partner. Talk to her like a friend too!

Different Listening Styles

You complain that women accuse you of not listening when you are. That's because we have different methods of absorbing what someone else is saying. We're more active listeners, really giving you our full attention when you speak. You tend to be more passive listeners, often paying us what I call "ear service," instead of fully absorbing what we say. We don't like that and many of you don't know why we complain so much about it. Let me educate you about listening skills.

The Importance of Listening

Effective listening means making an effort to hear what we say. It's not a facade of paying attention to humor us. We know your tricks! A good communicator must be a good listener. That means listening with the intent to hear what's said. If you're absorbed with your points and aren't concerned with hers, you're not communicating. You're listening to yourself speak. James shared an experience:

> I had a string of girlfriends before Jo-Ellen. I vaguely listened when they chattered about something or other, assuming women said nothing of interest to me. My buddies and I made fun of how women talk a lot of nonsense. We compared ways of tuning out. I still had those habits with Jo-Ellen and didn't pay her much attention. One night we went to a party with my buddies and their ladies. I went out back and was surprised when I returned to the main room that Jo-Ellen was talking avidly with a group of guys. Several told me later they envied me having a woman who could hold an intelligent conversation. They were amazed at how many things she had opinions about. Yet I never gave her a chance. After that I started listening more, really listening, and found out she has a lot to say that I enjoyed hearing, once I gave myself a chance. I sure learned something.

Good listening skills promote closeness between you and your partner. Instead of conversing with an attitude, think of it as a sharing experience. What we say is important to us, even if you don't agree. If we're important to you, take our thoughts seriously. Don't second-guess or trivialize them. You know that's unfair. We're not as predictable as you think. You may not listen because we speak about topics you find mundane—our friend's problems, shopping, an argument at work, what to wear. Hey, don't you care about her?! Take some interest in her life. If her thoughts are boring, why are you with her? Compromise on how much listening is reasonable.

Not listening is disrespectful. Sometimes we remind you of when you tuned out Mom's lectures as a child. She's not your mother! Her thoughts are as valuable as yours. You wouldn't like her ignoring you. If you learn to actively listen to what we want and follow through on your response to what we say, we'll give you an easier time. Don't be too stubborn. It doesn't get you much. Listening intently nourishes intimacy, making your connection stronger.

"Listen to Me" = Give Me Your Undivided Attention

Men and women listen differently and that's okay. But many of us don't always believe that you're legitimately listening, so we demand you do it our way. You may be happily working on your car when we talk to you; you continue fiddling; we get louder; you hear what we're saying, at least what you want to hear. But we complain you're not listening. What's up? You thought you were.

As long as words vaguely enter your ears, you're listening. According to Mary, good communication is "mutual understanding in both achieving a resolution and understanding what the other has to say. Attention and a lack of self-centeredness play a big role. Active listening is highly important. Eye contact and attentiveness are key." We're not satisfied without undivided attention. "Listen to us" can mean "look us straight in the eye when we speak." It means stop what you're doing and make us your only concern. Eye contact and having your attention is part of the connection that's important to us. I too get crazy when a guy doesn't pay attention according to my definition. You may not like doing it but it'll save you a lot of grief in the long run. Ginny said:

> When I'm talking to a guy, I want to talk to his face, not the back of his head or his chin. No matter what he says, it feels as though he's not listening if I can't see his eyes. Eyes say so much. Men hide a lot when they speak with their head turned, but eyes tell more. That's probably why they avoid looking at us when we're speaking of anything heavy. Men are fine with eye contact to get us into bed. But when we need to talk, they turn away. Most of them are cowards. A real man should face a woman who talks to him. If men would face us and get it over with, there'd be a lot fewer problems in relationships.

Why Women Can Be Long-Winded

We can go on and on once we start talking. It's hard to listen, especially when you construe it as criticism. I said earlier we face problems and you avoid them. Just as some of you fix cars, drains, or toasters, we like to fix the problems we see in our relationship.

Have you noticed that many of us repeat ourselves over and over? Ha ha! I'm sure you have. We don't do it to hear ourselves speak. If you don't respond we keep going. Blah, blah, blah, blah. We're scared of silence. You can sit and watch a game or fix something with a friend and not need to talk. We can't. I've had friends get crazy, asking what was wrong, because I was silent for a few minutes. We're not used to silence. Our insecurity talks when we press for a response. If we perceive something may be wrong, we need to talk. Ignoring us just gets us more frustrated, so we talk more.

THE DYNAMICS OF NAGGING

Nagging is the extreme of repeating ourselves. We often nag (repeat many times), if we don't get a satisfactory response. It worked as kids and it's hard to break the habit. We know some of you will begrudgingly give in if we harp enough. Most of us think we're repeating ourselves until we get an appropriate response. Lea told a coed group why she nags:

> I learned young if I wanted something, I had to ask for it over and over. Eventually I got listened to. I actually hate having to repeat myself with Ralph but often have no choice. If it was up to him he'd ignore everything I asked for. Last week he promised to fix the washing machine. I asked him when and he said "soon." After two days I asked again. Same answer. I needed to do a laundry so I asked more frequently. He called me a nag. Isn't there a word for a man who dodges his responsibility at home? He didn't do what he'd promised but I was the bad one. I repeat things because I get frustrated not getting a straight answer. If men would own up to their obligations, women would nag a lot less.

I relate to what Lea said. We ask questions and get grunts, nods, and evasive answers. It's frustrating, so we prod or repeat what we want until you do it. Give us straight answers when we ask for input, even if you don't care. If she asks about inviting your cousins for lunch or dinner, don't say it doesn't matter or either is fine. Show thought in your answer. If it concerns us, give it some importance. Be respectful of our need for your input.

WHY WE NAG

We want you to do something.

We're frustrated if you don't respond.

We want you to see our point, but you don't, or won't.

We can't get straight answers.

We want to control you.

Nagging is a bad habit most of us have had all our lives. Note the word *habit* and treat it as such. It takes time to break one that's been deeply ingrained, but you can help. At a peaceful time, explain to your partner how her nagging makes you feel, in a nice way. Follow my Commandments of Good Communication. Let her know how her constant harping wears your nerves thin. She may honestly not know the toll it takes. Spell it out in kind words, instead of jokes or barbs. Calmly explain that nagging doesn't work and just causes bad feelings. But, if she tries to control it, you'll try to give her more straight answers. Suggest other ways she can get through to you.

GETTING OFF THE PHONE

Talking on the phone gets tedious for those of you wanting to speak only when you have something to say. We're happy to get the connection of hearing your voice. Talking on the phone is an extension of gabfests with girlfriends. Since we like connections with friends and lovers, we don't relate to why many of you hate staying on the phone for longer than it takes to set a date, say hello, or share some news. We love idle conversation. You love getting off the phone quickly.

We feel neglected if you don't want to speak and you resent being kept on when you have things to do. Explain that it has nothing to do with her and you're willing to compromise but not be on the phone indefinitely. Decide what you can reasonably handle. Not all of you mind talking on the phone. But if you do, it can be worked out—off the phone.

MORE WALLS

This doesn't apply to all of you but I must address it. Something that frustrates us like crazy is how many of you put up walls when we're trying to talk about something serious. It's similar to the impenetrable walls I talked about in the last chapter, except it happens suddenly during a conversation. When we're troubled and you shut down as we talk, it's the most frustrating feeling imaginable. I've experienced this with boyfriends. Things were going smoothly and then a glitch occurred. I tried explaining the problem and felt those icy barbs I referred to creeping between us. Nothing I could say or do got through.

Guys, it's scary and painful to be with someone you care for deeply, who says he cares for you, and have him almost leave your reality while still being physically there. Our warm and loving guy becomes cold and seems heartless in an instant. When it's happened to me, I saw it coming but couldn't stop it. I'd always try talking but knew it was a lost cause. For those of you who do this, I know the signs—your voice gets almost robotic as you coldly enunciate your words. You become another person, a stranger. It feels as though your soul has left your body and only an empty shell is left. Trust me, I'm not being dramatic. Shari explained:

> When I talk to Bob when something bothers me, he often goes to another place. He's there yet he's not—like he's in another world where nothing I say is right. I never know what will trigger it. Sometimes I talk to him and he's fine. It's a relief but usually short-lived. I love him and he says he loves me but how many more of these moods or whatever they are can I handle? It wrings me out inside when he goes to that place. No matter how I try, nothing gets through to him then. We talk about it at other times. He vaguely knows he does it and said I shouldn't talk when it happens. That's not fair either. I shouldn't have to ignore what bothers me because he has a problem. I'll probably have to leave him.

The alienation caused by your refusal to listen with an open mind is painful beyond words. To be honest, the guys I've experienced it with seemed irrational when nothing I said was heard objectively. It has brought me to tears. When my last boyfriend did it, I was affected so badly that I began to scream in an effort to get through. And I have more tools for dealing with you than a lot of women. I wish I had better words to explain how frightening it feels to watch the man we care for become a stranger. When it passes, you may act as though nothing happened. We're emotionally drained.

What's the answer? I'm not sure. Some of you indicated that shutting down is a way of not dealing with being told what to do or that you're wrong. You may be afraid of getting hurt or not know how to handle a problem you can't solve so you turn inside for protection. The trouble is you're hurting someone you care about. Listen to her if she talks to you about it when it's not happening. Understand the impact when you do it. It's not good for you either—it alienates us and keeps you from resolving your problems.

Healthy Disagreements

We can compromise when one partner disagrees with the other. The key to ironing out differences is respecting each other, and acknowledging that each has a right to disagree with the other. This doesn't mean that you will always reach an agreement. It's okay if you don't always think alike.

BENEFITS OF DISAGREEMENTS/FIGHTING

You're known for avoiding confrontations at all costs. We're known for provoking. Some of you brag that you've never had a fight with your partner. That doesn't mean there's no trouble. Verbal confrontations are healthy for relationships. Disagreeing is normal. The more people are together, the more potential there is to disagree. Friends fight. Families fight. Lovers fight. We fight differently. Your fights with men may be louder. We sometimes fight dirty using tears and emotional maneuvers to create guilt.

Couples who never fight rarely resolve problems. Bringing problems into the open can clear bad feelings. Disagreements don't have to be mean or loud. If you treat each other's feelings with respect, you can have a stronger relationship. After any disagreement, forgive.

Even if you know you were right, apologize for making her feel bad. Remember compassion. You don't have to apologize for your actions if you believe you did nothing wrong, but say you're sorry about how it makes her feel. Bonus: Making up can be very sweet!

I believe healthy disagreements increase trust. If we tiptoe around issues, resentment brews. Things may seem peaceful but one of you may have unspoken anger and eventually the other may discover it in an unpleasant way—like erupting over something trivial. It's harder to trust if you wonder what hasn't been said. My friends/boyfriends don't always like what I say but they appreciate my expressing something that bothers me. They know I have no hidden resentment. After we talk I let it go. Sometimes what I say results in an argument but we get through it and trust each other more because we say what we think—the truth.

Saying "Nothing is wrong" is dishonest. Don't be afraid to tell the truth or argue. Keep respect in the picture. Express yourself or disagree to resolve situations, not to score the winning point. If you're willing to sincerely listen to her point of view, you'll have a more solid relationship. Alan said:

> I used to think of fighting with a woman as a lose/lose situation. It seemed hopeless to get her to see my point. If I did, there'd be tears. My wife and I went to counseling and we began fighting during sessions. Instead of getting out of control, we got our points across and often found a solution. I learned a lot about my wife during our disagreements. I've stopped thinking of them as fights because we don't yell—we just tell each other things that bother us and try talking it out. We don't always agree but we've learned to accept that we're entitled to think differently about things. Our marriage is more solid.

If you sense she's upset, she may imitate you at first by saying "Nothing is wrong." Let her know you care and sincerely want to know what's troubling her (even if it's the last thing you want to know). Then it can be dealt with and you can move on. We do want you to know what's bothering us but sometimes need to know you care enough to pull it out of us. Be man enough to pull hard. Communication solves problems and we know you love fixing things!

WORKING ON PROBLEMS

I can't repeat enough the importance of respecting each other's right to an opinion. This enables you to work together to find solutions for problems. When things are going well, sit in a relaxed environment and discuss your options for when problems come up. Explain nicely what gets you most riled during an argument. Ask her to do the same. If you can share and explain, rather than criticize and blame, more cooperation can develop. Don't be too defensive about what she shares. That only hurts communication. Learn to ask questions like, "How can we work together to get things straight?" And work together! Get used to being open-minded as you practice communication skills. Greg said:

> *Zena and I are very different. We get along most of the time but avoid talking about things that might cause a problem. Then Zena came to me and asked me to sit down. I thought, "Uh oh, she's gonna dump me." But she didn't. She did ask how I'd like to talk about things that are important to the growth of our relationship. She disagreed with some of my ways and wanted me to know. My first reaction was to clam up but I like Zena a lot and want to stay with her. We talked about fights we'd had in other relationships and what bothered us about disagreements. I warned her I can lose my temper which was why I avoided fights. She asked if it was okay for her to leave the room if I did. Our disagreements are more peaceful than in the past because we set up ground rules. We don't want to hurt each other so we're working together.*

Setting ground rules is effective. Talk about what annoys you about your disagreements when you're on good terms. As you get to know each other, you'll learn each other's pattern of handling disagreements. One of you may shout (you?). One may need to go into graphic details that aren't necessary (her?). Each of you has at least some annoying pattern or attitude for holding your own in a disagreement, even if you don't recognize your own foibles. Rather than push each other's buttons, be straight about what annoys you and encourage her to be straight with you. Talk during peaceful times. Then you can be more sensitive about what escalates problems.

Connection Tip

> When you have a disagreement, focus on the issues or situation, not on her personally. "IT—not you—makes me unhappy."

Take a time-out if an argument goes nowhere. Going in circles to convince each other and getting more riled up merit taking a breather. Acknowledge that space is needed. Of course, we may protest. We like resolving things right away—even issues that need time. It's our nature to talk until you get it, often out of fear. We're scared you'll leave if you're angry, so we want things to be okay before we separate from you. Reassure her that the problem can and will eventually be worked out so she's comfortable allowing space to cool down and think.

My Ten Commandments of Communication works during disagreements. Stick to your point. Don't allow anger to make you digress to other issues that bother you. If we get on your case about something, don't attack in defense or it can escalate into an unnecessary full-fledged battle. Solving relationship problems involves two. If your partner has difficulty cooperating, you'll need the patience of two. Communicating as a team gives you the best chance of having a healthy, successful relationship.

Couples seem to communicate well in the beginning. When we're just getting to know each other, we're anxious to talk and make a good impression. Once it's a relationship, the need can dissipate fast. Some of you say that you talk at work and want quiet at home. You'd love to stop thinking altogether if you could! But we need conversations with you that aren't just by rote. We need to know you're listening—it helps cement the connection we crave. Good interaction out of bed can carry over into bed. Developing playful banter and interesting dialogue will put her in a better mood for more fun activities.

7 *Programmed Agendas: Upgrading Expectations*

You've dated for six months and she's hinting for commitment. You just want to have fun. Going to a wedding last week didn't help. Now a friend has a baby and she gets a funny look when she sees it. You've told her women are too fixated on commitment and she should lighten up. You know her friends make it worse. She says you're too fixated on basic needs like sex, food, and partying and she knows your friends make it worse. Why can't women relax and have fun? Why do they have those expectations? You're sure your friends are right. You should be just going for lots of fun and sex. Why does she keep saying your friends have the wrong expectations? They have none! ∼

Both sexes have agendas about relationships. Yours might be more subtle. In the beginning, women, the pleasing-by-nature sex, may go out of their way to meet your needs, so relationships often start out in your favor. We're on good behavior at first, especially to prove we'd make a good partner. As time passes, many of us push for commitment.

Unrealistic Expectations
I've explained where our needs come from. Our agendas are programmed like yours are. Marriage and children are still heralded as our ultimate goal. Trust me, they're potent! Some of us are trying to change but it's hard to

break lifetime habits. You're connected to many things we think we need to be happy. It's not our fault, nor yours. It's just the way it is.

STACKED AGENDAS

I believe that women often approach dating with a stacked deck. You see early dating as an opportunity to have fun, and maybe have sex. We may evaluate you as a potential partner so it's hard to relax and just have fun. Being on a mission to find a provider adds pressure from the get-go. Our needs aren't compatible.

Many of us never learned to be independent. Had you been brought up as many of us were, you'd have agendas too. If we're told to go to college to get our MRS. degree, if we're taught we're not whole people without a man, if we believe we're not attractive until you tell us we are, how can we separate you from our happiness? It wasn't our choice to make you so important. It's been drummed into our heads. Patti explained her dilemma:

> I'm vice president of a decent-sized corporation and worked hard to get here. Yet my whole adult life feels like it's been one big question—"When are you going to get a man and get married?" My mom is proud of me on one level but always says my real success will be marriage. I hate seeing family because I always get the question. I've been fighting it but it scares me that I do always watch for a good partner. I'm ashamed that I've bought the indoctrination. With everything I do, no matter how much I act like I don't need a man, I want one very badly. I still have a better feeling about myself when I'm in a relationship. It's scary. I can't separate whether I want a man for them or for me. Either way, it sucks!

Women got therapy and an ability to talk about problems. You guys got independence. It frightens me how many women still concentrate their self-help/therapy on finding a man. Successful, intelligent women in my classes say they aren't happy without one. Check out all the books on how to find and keep you. Do you still wonder why we date you with our needs hanging out? We continue trying to find "Mr. Right," and if we can't find him, we'll settle for "Mr. Not Too Wrong" and try revamping him to fit the mold.

Agenda-Makers

Our expectations can get numerous and specific. I know they drive you crazy. We often drive ourselves crazy too! But where do they come from? Other women. We gather together, decide what relationships should or shouldn't have, and mandate rules. Fair? No way! Many of us discuss and overanalyze; we feed each other's anger. We pick and choose what suits us. We gang up on you in private if we're angry at not getting what WE think relationships should be. We reinforce each other's need for you, and expect you to provide what WE think you should. I agree that's totally unfair.

Before you get too indignant, I'll point out that you do it too. Guys set standards for how a woman should look and act. You say your friends can be just as hard on us when it comes to our appearance and expectations of what we should do for you. Guys create their own standards. You get judged and sentenced by juries of women who collectively set unfair standards for relationships. Ned said:

> It was delightful when Susan and I first met. We fell into an easy rhythm of doing things together. After four months I saw a subtle change. She wanted routines and to see each other more. I got more personal questions about my job and feelings about family. I almost withdrew as I've done before. Instead I asked what was going on. She was embarrassed. Said her cousin and friends had been pushing her to think about the future. I asked what she wanted. She cried and said nobody cared what she wanted. Her family treated her like a loser because I hadn't committed. It was only four months! Susan liked our relationship but the pressure was getting to her. I said I liked her but it was too soon to commit. I was willing to keep going and see if our relationship could grow, as long as that happened just between us, not a conspiracy by friends and family. We're both happy again. I feel sorry for Susan—feeling so much pressure to do what others say as law.

If you're feeling pressure, I suggest both of you put your expectations on the table. Come on. You have them too—maybe yours are great sex and basic comforts. Speak without an attitude. Make it a conversation. Without getting angry or rebellious, use the skills in Chapter 6 to communicate how you feel and what you'd like. State your view in a friendly way. Don't criticize her for having an agenda. Use compassion to understand why she needs certain commitments, but say it's making you uncomfortable. Try compromising. I doubt she'll just let go of her agenda but she might ease up a bit. Or, she might not be right for you.

Not all of us are mercenary or bent on finding a lifetime partner. Once in a relationship, I believe what we need from each other is more balanced. You may see your needs as less demanding because you haven't understood ours before. Rod said, "Men are simple creatures. Give them love, sex, affection, and some space and a woman can make almost any man happy." We don't need more than that. Give us affection, compliments, intimacy, connect to us with little things, and listen to what we're saying if you want to make us happy. Our needs take no more effort than yours. They're just different.

DIFFERENT AGENDAS FOR SEX

Often we have different agendas in bed. You may want sex for physical relief. If it's with someone you like a lot—even better! We often have sex to feel loved. We take your tenderness, sweet words, and enthusiasm too seriously. You may mean them at the moment. We may want them to be permanent. Many of us think that you'll stay if we have sex. You know the deal on that one too. I asked men and women why they have sex. More of our reasons were tied to being loved, needing affection, or getting closer, though horniness was important too. Although many of you acknowledged that sex with a woman you love is the best, your focus was more on physical pleasure than ours.

Consistent with our program, we focus more on you than you are on us. We often make you more important than sex itself. It's harder for us to separate sex and love. We (and our friends) read into every passionate kiss, every tender touch, and every loving look. The "Ooo, that orgasm felt great" response gets interpreted as "I'm crazy about you." Be careful how thickly you lay it on when you're not sure how you feel. We take everything you do in bed personally. Sex can create pressure. Her expectations of you can change to thinking of you as a guy she might marry because of your passionate response to an orgasm.

 Connection Tip

Give her a hug once in a while, just because.

The Attraction of Security

You complain that some women act as though your bank account is more important than who you are and that you should bring a resume on a date for the personal questions. We date like we shop and check you out like a commodity. If you don't have good partner potential, you may be history. I'm completely on your side if you're thinking we have convoluted values about security. But I've been on the other side and know how strong the pressure is. It's scary thinking that we're not a whole person without you. Family members *still* ask who will take care of me when I'm old if I don't get married. Do any of you get asked that?

Judging You Quickly

Lou asked in a men's class, "How can women make snap judgments about me?" "Why don't they get to know me better?" chimed Bert. Many guys said we drop you in a flash if you don't meet our initial criteria. We're not that bad. But when agendas are strong and pressure to meet them stronger, we choose to only go out with a potentially good partner. Just as we don't try on clothing that's not exactly what we want, some of us don't waste time if you don't fit our picture.

But you're quick to judge too. You admit making instant judgments based on appearance. If our appearance doesn't fit your agenda, you won't waste time talking. Gary admitted:

> I don't like women's questions—about my profession; whether I pay alimony or child support; do I want children. I had it in my head that women were the shallow ones until I hung with some single friends. They talked about women they'd met and analyzed every

inch of their bodies. One stopped seeing a woman because her breasts were too small. One dropped a woman because he thought he could find someone thinner. I heard little about what they thought of them as people. It's a guy thing I guess—choose a woman by looks. We check out their bodies, hair, eyes, and more. We learned to judge them by hanging together. We discuss what's attractive and avoid what other guys make fun of. Women learned to look for security and marriage stuff from their friends. We're all shallow!

What we think we need is reinforced by those close to us. Your ability to earn a living is highlighted when friends and loved ones check out who we're dating. We get asked regularly, "What does he do for a living?" If our guy doesn't have a job they perceive as appropriate, we see an attitude and feel like a loser. Unfortunately, many folks act more concerned with the financial status of our potential mate than what kind of person he is. Since we're programmed to please, many of us pursue men with qualities we're told are essential. Please be aware of what you put out. I've found that many men who complain about how mercenary women are use cars and other signs of money to lure them. Once you see your worth apart from your possessions, more women will too!

Feminine Double Standards

Women say they want to be treated equally. We bitch about double standards. We whine about not having equal opportunities. We fight for equitable salaries. Some of us say we don't need help and rebel if you hold a door. Yet some will ditch you if you don't buy them dinner.

I ask women in my classes what that makes them besides hypocrites. What are we saying? That we want equal rights when it suits us? That you can't use double standards but we can? We're used to you paying our way. It makes us feel special and we don't want to lose that. Many of you aren't comfortable having us pay either. Few men I date let me kick in for the check, but I offer. Women with a more equitable attitude about dating agree with me. Those who want to be taken out, receive gifts, get wined and dined, and be treated for everything scoff at my words. I was horrified when Gail described a dating experience at her summer-share:

> *I met Joseph in the Hamptons. The main social activity was going to parties in people's homes or at clubs. We'd go to them together every weekend. I was attracted to him and we'd make out when he took me home. After six weeks, he initiated sex. I was furious and told him how dare he expect me to sleep with him when he hadn't bought me dinner yet.*

I wanted to ask her if she was a prostitute, since she'd sleep with a guy if he bought dinner. Many of you expressed anger at women who seem almost mercenary. I agree. Our actions may say we'll take equality when it's in our favor. Many women are accustomed to an expensive lifestyle and want a guy to accommodate them. Some of you would be happy with one who shared your lifestyle interests. If you want a partner who values you before your wallet, don't stick around with one who doesn't, unless the sex is worth it. She won't change if she falls in love. Her values will haunt you as she pushes you to advance in your career. Find a woman who's on the same wavelength as you. We're out there!

Marry Me, Marry Me/Tick, Tick, Tick

I can't emphasize strongly enough how marriage is heralded as our dream. While you played with trucks and balls as a kid, we made believe we were getting married. I knew a woman who was obsessed with getting married—but not because she wanted a guy to share her life with. She'd planned her wedding since childhood. Every guy she dated endured scrutiny about getting married. She blew off some great ones who wouldn't commit fast enough and finally latched onto a guy she'd referred to as a nerd. She had her wedding and now tries to convince herself it was worth it. A wedding seems enticing if we've idealized it our whole life.

You're taught that marriage is part of your life. We're taught it defines ours. Getting married shows you want us, so we feel worthy. Some woman will marry almost anyone, even if it's likely to end in divorce, just to say they've been married. Getting married makes our mothers happy. As we get older, pressure to get married starts. Although times are changing, many of us still feel the stigma of "old maid" hanging over our heads. Some of you are prodded by mothers who want grandchildren, but most of you don't get the same pressure.

The biological clock has a huge effect on our need for you. This is very important for you to understand. We have no right to judge a woman for wanting a child, even if it's an obsession. How can we pass judgment if she's scared her time is running out? You can always marry a younger woman, but as we get older, there's less chance to conceive. Some women panic if they want a child and there's no potential father. Doctors say our desire to bear children is biological, not just societal pressure. When our clock is counting down, we look hard for a husband. Alison said:

> I want a baby so badly. I always bought the dream that I'd meet the guy for me, get married, and have children. Well, I'm thirty-six and getting scared. I used to be relaxed about marriage. But as I hear of women not being able to conceive as they get older, I become more on the look-out for a husband. My brother tells me to lighten up but he can't talk. He's dating women in their twenties. Forget the dream. I don't care as much about him fitting my needs. A nice guy who wants children will do now. I sound awful, don't I?

Many women feel like Alison. I have tremendous compassion for those desperate for a child. Although we can have babies in our forties, it's more of a crapshoot to wait until the clock has almost ticked out. I encourage women to face that marrying for a baby probably won't make them happy; they may not have children; hunting for a sperm donor won't create a healthy family. I've advised therapy for coping. I wish there was a reasonable solution. Be compassionate and patient with women who are dying for a baby, even if you don't want one. It's a sad situation, with no happy answer. Just try to be clear about what you want, even if she doesn't like it.

Mr. Fix-Its

We're not the only fix-its in a relationship. Some of you may take on our problems. Are you subconsciously attracted to a helpless woman who offers you a chance to be a man? Finding one to renovate is no better than our trying to fix you. If you don't want to be our Prince Charming, don't look for Eliza Doolittle.

Damaged Women

You bring past problems into a relationship. We do too. Women with problems can stimulate some of you to get out your toolbox and patch their damage. Many of you said you fall for women who seem helpless. Vulnerability motivates you to don your knight in shining armor suit, protect them, and fix their lives. STOP! Paul was ashamed when he told a class:

> I met Shea in a bar. She was sweet and helpless, saying men had treated her badly in the past. She was struggling to make something of her life. I admired her determination and we began dating. I admit I liked feeling needed. But she became a pest, interrupting me at work. I asked her to stop but she'd cry—and I'd weaken. She did nothing to help herself. She had excuses instead of a job. I loaned her money but she'd want more. I eventually understood why men haven't treated her right. I wanted to shake her—tell her to leave me alone—get her life together. I've been attracted to women like this before. Growing up I was the youngest and always felt useless. I like helping. But I'm trying to stop dating needy women—I'm never happy after the first few weeks of taking care of them.

You say you like helping us and often end up angry if you don't get the eternal gratitude you crave. Neither sex should choose a partner they have to fix. Your need to "be the man" for a woman with serious problems won't work. It makes you feel important, for a while. Do volunteer work for charity if you need a project. You might meet a nice woman there.

Romantic Tip

Occasionally leave a Post-It note on her mirror or fridge that starts off, "One reason I like (love) you is . . ." Be specific about something she does that brightens your life.

HEALTHY WOMEN

Set your sights on a healthy partner. Why take responsibility for someone else's life? We may not need specific things, but will appreciate your presence. I consider myself reasonably healthy and can take care of myself. But I love getting support from a guy I'm seeing. We can all use it.

Very needy women drain you with demands. You complain you have to call too much, listen to problems, build her low self-esteem, etc. Hey guys, both sexes can be attracted to someone who needs us. It makes us feel important and creates a false sense of security that they'll stay. But it rarely makes us happy. It's lovely when someone is with you because they want to be, not have to be. Support a partner by being there, providing compassion, and giving great hugs. You can't shield her from life. Kent told a group:

> *I was a professional lady-fixer for years. The more she needed, the more I plunged into her life, ready to show her a better way. Each girlfriend stuck around until she tired of me, or I got tired of being drained by her problems. I'll always be grateful to a friend who saw my pattern and yelled at me. She pushed me to make an effort to attract women without serious problems. I realized I felt safer with ones who did and became determined to find my safety in a good woman. When I met Sarah, I got scared. She had her life together and I didn't know where I'd fit in. With my friend's encouragement, I used the energy I used to give women to work on my confidence. Sarah and I have been together for a year and I've never been happier. I still get insecure at times but that's life. At least I'm happy!*

I implore you to put energy into developing a friendship with a woman who seems right for you. When your lover is also your good friend, the relationship has a much better shot at peaceful longevity.

It comes in handy during times when one of you needs support. You're notorious for disappearing when we need you most—during an illness; a death; a career change, etc. Even if you hate hospitals or funerals, force yourself to be there for us. Even if the choice we're making will change your routine or income, let us know we have your support. Support is one of the greatest gifts you can give us.

Autonomy versus Possessiveness

When you want a night with the guys, why do many of us act like we'll be lost or ask "What will I do?" When you need time to yourself, why can't we find something to do instead of making you feel guilty? You're often frustrated by a partner's inability to amuse herself or cope if you don't spend all your time with her. It's our programs again. Many of us don't know how to function happily on our own. We haven't learned to enjoy our own company.

Our Fun versus Your Fun

Why can't we find things to do? As girls, we may not have learned to have the kind of fun you did. Our activities didn't encourage bonding. You had more opportunities to play team sports and do activities with fewer boundaries. You didn't stay as clean and quiet. Your play environment was more fun. We have more intimate friendships than most of you, but there's no female equivalent of male bonding.

When women get together with friends, most of us discuss work, problems with friends, or our primary topic of conversation—you. We talk about our current guy—where to find one—anger toward you—frustration without you. You can be playful or get stupid with your friends. Many of us don't know how to have that kind of fun. Our friends can be more of a sympathetic ear than a playmate. Some women do go out drinking and carousing like many of you. More of us prefer being with a guy for fun.

While you shared sports and lively activities as kids, we played quietly. As a teen you bonded through sports, drinking, being stupid together, etc. My teen friends and I spent our time working on our appearance or looking for a boyfriend. Many of you still have fun with your friends. Many of us don't have a foundation for truly enjoying a "girls' night out." Being with you is sweeter. We're notorious for ignoring friends if we're seeing someone. If we're in a relationship, our need for friends can diminish, except when we need to complain.

Do you give up friends when you're in a relationship? I bet you don't. You've said that going out with friends is a time for fun. You share activities that most women don't: sports—playing or going to games, and watching them at home or in a bar; playing cards; drinking; going to hear live music; other fun activities. When many of us go out, we're preoccupied with meeting men. You told me you're usually not looking to meet women on nights out with the guys. You enjoy doing things you may not get to do with us. Barry said:

> I felt superior to my sister when I was growing up. I can't remember when she wasn't obsessed with boys. She'd sit with friends, fixing each other's hair, talking about who to attract. I'm older yet her boy thing started before I stopped running from girls. Girls always chased me since I was tall and looked older but I wasn't interested—my friends were more fun. She's never stopped making men the center of her world. I've talked to her but don't think she knows what else to do. If I hadn't been exposed to my sister, I'd have less patience with my girlfriend, who's learning to enjoy her autonomy more.

Many of you expressed dismay about how much time we want with you. It's not as easy for us to have fun. Getting drunk has a stigma for women. You act loud and silly. It's not ladylike. If we do what's normal for you we may be judged as sluts, unfeminine, etc. So most of our socializing revolves around you—analyzing you, complaining about you, hunting for you, etc. Too many of us only go places with potential to meet men. We weren't taught to enjoy each other's company or to have a life. Since being with friends isn't nearly as much fun as what you do, we put all our eggs in your basket.

Fighting for Space

If we don't need it, we have a hard time understanding your need for time without us and often take it personally. Since many of us would rather be with you, your need to spend time without us can make us insecure. We get touchy about things that come across as macho. Guy activities push our buttons. Going out drinking with friends or getting involved with sports represents our being excluded.

What happened to autonomy? Those of you in a relationship ask "Do we have to be like one person all the time?" Emphatically, "No!" A relationship where both partners maintain their autonomy is the best. I encourage women to get a life. How can you keep your sanity and autonomy? Explain to her: Your need to do things without her has nothing to do with your feelings nor enjoyment of her company; you enjoy going out with friends; enjoying space doesn't mean she's less important to you. Encourage her to develop her own interests. When she does something on her own, tell her how attractive it is. That may encourage her! You can keep your identity in a relationship. Jamel called after a workshop:

> Dee had a problem if I'd go out without her. I'd get mad and do what I wanted—she'd get upset and say I didn't love her. After your workshop, I asked about her childhood friendships. Dee saw her younger years as happy but I didn't hear enthusiasm about friends. Playing with dolls and acting out dreams of meeting Prince Charming wasn't the fun my friends had. As a teen she was always looking for guys. Other activities were shopping, gossiping with friends, and going to parties to meet guys. I had my share of meeting girls but my friends did crazy things that were even more fun. I now understand why she has a hard time when I go out. Her activities with friends now are mainly shopping and conversations. I've been patient with Dee and explained what you told us. She understands more why I go with friends and why she'd rather be with me. We're trying to compromise. I've been encouraging her to take a class or join a group that might interest her. She's trying.

If your partner balks at your doing things without her, don't get defensive or fight. If she hates your going bowling and it's something you enjoy, go without guilt. It's her problem, not yours. You shouldn't have to apologize for going. Say that you're sorry it bothers her but you have a right to your own activities, just as she can have hers. Don't try finding something for her to do unless she'd like help. Acknowledge that she's lonely when you're out—you hate knowing it but have a right to your activity. Let compassion for her unhappiness and inability to amuse herself motivate your tolerance, even if you think she's foolish and should cope. David said, "I've tried to install a regular schedule with the woman I'm seeing. She knows when we're getting together and I give her regular phone calls."

 Romantic Tip

Tell her how she's gotten sexier the more you know her, and why you're lucky to have her.

WATCHING SPORTS

Our emotional reaction to sports may seem over the top. We associate it with exclusion, so we can get sensitive when you mention wanting to watch a game. The bottom line is that a majority of us would be happy if you'd give us a good dose of the attention/affection we love when it doesn't interfere with your activity.

You can watch sports on TV with your partner around without alienating her. She may personalize and assume she doesn't mean as much as the game. Since we need to know you care, some affection can offset ignoring us when you're watching. Relationships and sports can mix. It may not always be perfect but I bet most of you will enjoy your games more. Here are five tips for enjoying sports without alienating your partner:

1. *Have patience.* Getting annoyed if she balks won't help. Understanding why it may bother her can motivate you to make an effort to get her more comfortable with your interest in sports.

2. *Explain some basics of the game.* Many women don't like sports because we don't understand them. Offer to explain how the game works. Although she might act "girlie" when listening, give it a shot if she shows interest. It might be fun!

3. *Make plans to do something with her before or after a game.* If it's on later in the day, go for brunch before. If it's early, plan to go out for dinner, rent a movie and snuggle, or do something else she likes after the game or the next evening. We need to feel that time with us is important to you.

4. *Give her affection during breaks.* A kiss, some hugs, tender caresses, and other small actions to cement your connection will go far in making her more relaxed. She may come to like when you're watching a game if she knows she'll get some goodies when you do.

5. *Let her know you appreciate her accepting your interest in sports.* For many of us, being considerate about sports is something we need to work at. Acknowledging that you know it's not easy for her and you appreciate her consideration may make her feel better about doing it.

If you care about your partner and have compassion about why it bothers her so much, you can make her feel better and watch a game in reasonable peace. Lenny shared with a support group:

The biggest cause of static between Wendy and me was ball games. When we first dated, she said she didn't mind and sometimes watched with me. As we got serious, she said we should do things we both liked. Living together was worse. After hearing you and understanding her point of view at least somewhat, I tried using the compassion you recommended. It's working. I say I love her more. Attention definitely made a difference. When the guys join me on a Sunday, I take Wendy for dinner after. Now they join us with their girlfriends—they've seen a difference too. Last Sunday I made love to Wendy during half time and didn't mind missing some of the second half. She liked that. I talk to her about why I enjoy sports. She's relaxing and making plans with friends instead of sitting home sulking. Sometimes she'll read while I watch and we snuggle. I used to rebel about giving attention—I resented her attitude. Now I understand she wasn't trying to be controlling, and don't mind. She likes Sundays more because we have fun when the game's not on.

Are you so obsessed with sports that it dominates your life? That's not good for a relationship or for yourself. Also, be aware of how annoying your buddies may be to her if they join you. Women complain that their men expect them to play waitress during the game to a bunch of loud, drunken guys. No wonder your watching games gets a bad rep among women.

To Commit—Or Not to Commit

Sooner or later she's going to push for commitment. That's reality and she has a right to want it. You have a right not to. Outside pressure tells us we should get a commitment after some point. Many of us don't evaluate nearly as much as you do when considering a long-term partner. As long as a guy meets certain criteria, we're less fussy about others. You, on the other hand, often put a woman you're considering for commitment through a silent scrutiny that few of us can pass. Again our needs are different.

Fear of Commitment

Committing to marriage, or living together, can be scary. While fear of getting hurt is there, other factors influence your avoiding that final "I will." Commitment can shift responsibility to you as a traditional breadwinner. Thinking of kids increases pressure. You may fear feeling claustrophobic or stuck. Many of you wonder if you'll meet someone better. If she's anxious to get married you also may worry that she's settling for you. Keep it in perspective. It's normal to have doubts, but don't let them keep you from committing to a woman you see as a good partner. You'll never find perfection. Omar had doubts:

> I was with Debbie almost two years. We got along well and I was attracted to everything about her. Then she started bringing up the "C" word—commitment. Friends warned me about it. I always assumed I'd get married and liked the idea. But things my friends said made commitment something to automatically run from. I avoided discussions. Debbie said at that point I should know how I

felt about her. She was in love with me and wanted to work toward marriage. I loved her too but panicked. All my friends' jokes and warnings about commitment replayed in my head. I refused to discuss it and she gave me an ultimatum. Friends were indignant so we broke up. After a month I was miserable and saw having Debbie in my life was good. I told my friends to shut up and asked for a second chance. We're getting married next year. I have time to acclimate myself to being married. We'll live together as a transition. I'm grateful I didn't lose the best part of my life.

Are you scared that if you commit, she'll be less tolerant of what she's accepted in you. You may worry you'll lose your space or a special chair or a place that's your comfort zone might have to go. Your life may feel more restricted if it's shared. You may like being able to go home if one of you is in a bad mood. I relate to all of these. When we're used to life one way, it's hard to adapt it 100 percent for anyone. Eighty percent still gives me breathing room if he goes home sometimes. Try that on for size before making it 100 percent. Ease into it slowly, talk about doubts, and see if it can work first.

 Which is worse?

Losing her or losing your freedom? List at least five things you might lose for each. Weigh each list to decide which is worse. Do you want to live without her?

WAITING FOR PERFECTION

Are you looking for perfection? If you never find it, you're safe from commitment. Think about that. Your concerns about whether or not she's right for you can focus too much on specific elements instead of keeping all the reasons you're with her in perspective. She may have all this but is missing one piece, so you hesitate or wait for better. Nobody is perfect—it's nearly impossible for someone to have every quality you'd like. Decide what's most important in a partner and focus on getting someone with those qualities. *Your* agendas can be more rigid once you decide it's time to settle down. Many of you have said you know exactly what you want in a long-term partner. Lighten up! I've spoken with too many guys who left a woman they were falling in love with because she was missing criteria. Chad said:

> I used to do marathon dating. When I hit my thirties safe sex issues made me feel it was time to settle down. I met great women but was compelled to find my Ms. Right. If I committed to one, she had to have everything so I kept searching. When I met Daisy I was intrigued. She was different from others I'd dated but it felt good. I did a checklist. She wasn't my dream woman so I pulled back—I didn't want to like her too much if she didn't fit my bill. I dated other women but thought about Daisy. It confused me. My sister asked what happened between us and I told her. She laughed, saying men can be stupid. Daisy made me happy. Wasn't that key? I guess commitment is permanent so I put pressure on myself to choose the right partner. Daisy and I are now living together and I've never been happier. Every day I'm more certain I made the right choice. Had I waited for what I thought was the ideal Ms. Right, I'd have missed the real one.

Commitment doesn't have to be all or nothing. Compromise. Ease into it slowly, IF you believe she may be right for you. Spend more time with her gradually so you can try it on for comfort. Be honest about your fear of losing your space. See how she responds. If she's willing to work with you, there's a great chance of it working. Set a time limit of at least three months to a year to think about commitment and ask her not to speak of it until the deadline. At that point if you're not sure, stop seeing her. You may change your mind if you miss her enough. You may not.

8

UPGRADING YOUR APPEAL: MAXIMIZING YOUR ATTRACTIVENESS TO WOMEN

You meet a guy whose looks aren't nearly as good as you think yours are with a girlfriend more attractive than any you've had. You wonder if he's rich or has a ten-inch penis. Later you learn he just makes an average living. You still wonder about his penis. She seems truly happy with him. You wonder what's so special about him that attracts such a woman. "What's wrong with me?" you think. You wonder if you'll ever figure out how to attract the women you'd really like. Where's your fairy godmother when you need her?! ~

You can increase your chances of making a good impression on women. There's no pat answer for what we look for in a man. Some of us are more into looks or money than others are. Some need an intellectual connection. Some (no offense) are desperate for a husband and will settle for anyone. There are things you can work on that affect how we perceive you. I've asked women what attracts them or puts them off.

Good Grooming Goes a Long Way

"Why do some women insist on grooming me like I was a pet?" you ask. She finds you attractive enough at first. But as the initial rush calms, she tries to change your appearance. Many of us see you as clay waiting to be molded. Often what we recommend will do you more good than harm. Of course it's not fair to expect you to change your grooming habits and style of dress. But get real! Some of you have none. A little more style won't hurt you!

SHE DOESN'T HAVE TO KNOW:
You didn't shower today.
Your ex bought the shirt you're wearing.
You can't remember when you washed your sheets.
You trim hair in places that aren't on your head.

IMAGE CONSULTANTS

Our overall appearance can shout what we think of ourselves. If you look as though you don't care about how you look, it can be translated as not thinking much of yourself. An effort to be neat and clean, in clothes that fit, tells the world you have a good self-image. We're all attracted to people who look like they care about their appearance.

No matter what you look like, the right clothes and a good haircut can make you look better. Find a style you feel good in. Neat and clean is more attractive than just throwing on clothes without caring. Many men who are overweight, short, bald (not by choice) or who don't have the greatest face can have a nicer appearance in clothes that are neat, stylish and fit properly. Get clothes that enhance, not detract from your appearance.

Ask female friends or people in stores for suggestions. You don't have to dress up. To me, well-fitted jeans and a clean T-shirt are the sexiest attire. But I see guys in jeans that hang in the wrong places and T-shirts with stains—what a turnoff! So you hate shopping—it's worth an effort to find clothes that fit well. I had a boyfriend who wore poorly fitting unstylish jeans—shopping made him hyperventilate so he never tried them on. When he succumbed to going shopping with me and got several pairs that fit great, he admitted feeling better about himself. He also loved my reaction. Looking as if you paid attention to your appearance is attractive. Rick said:

> *I didn't like Margie interfering with how I looked. Women complain we criticize their weight and such so I rebelled at anything she said. She suggested someone to cut my hair—that she go shopping with me—new sheets. No way! It felt like she wasn't happy with me. I complained to my sister who asked what was so terrible. I accused her of ganging up with Margie but she said she'd always*

wanted to suggest things but it wasn't her place. Why didn't I try something new? So I got a haircut and clothes Margie chose. I was surprised how many people at work noticed and complimented me. Even Margie gives me more attention. It does make me feel better about myself. I admit having new sheets so I can change them more often is nice too. I won't tell Margie, but she was right.

Many of you like our input. The most common stuff we try to change is easier than what you expect from us. Some of you push us to lose weight, wear sexier clothing, and look youthful, which are hard. We may suggest a haircut, clothes, and simple things that improve your appearance dramatically. They can make you more attractive to everyone.

GOOD HYGIENE

Paula said what frustrates her most about men is "not keeping their hygiene up to par." Women complain you can be pigs. Although many of you don't deserve the bad rap, we tend to be more fastidious. You have a reputation for being less concerned about changing underwear as regularly; not changing sheets or doing laundry as often; not caring about your clothes as much; not bathing as much. We know that you're not all like this, but we're sensitive. Lily pointed out:

I accept that most women will be more meticulous than most men. But men can be gross. I've dated some who thought taking a shower every two or three days was being meticulous. Most men aren't overtly dirty, but I get turned off when a man smells himself or his underwear to decide whether to shower or change clothes. They do that. Women can be picky to an extreme about being clean but a man who shows no interest in grooming is hard to take. When I meet a man, I pay attention to his attitude about his habits.

Some of you are self-acknowledged pigs and think it's funny if we cringe when you wear the same underwear for days. Although you have a right to your own habits, you're better off keeping untidy ones to yourself. You complain that some of us are over the top with standards. Billy said:

Just because my girlfriend showers every morning, doesn't mean I have to. I'm not a pig. I do things on a looser schedule. I shower most days but not on schedule. When I stay over, she's snotty in the morning if she asks if I'm going to shower and I say "no." She makes faces. I've learned if I say I'll shower at home, she leaves me alone. I shower when I'm dirty, but many don't accept that. So I let them think I'm doing more. They get too fussy.

If you want to make a good impression on a woman you're intimate with, especially at the beginning, don't tell her all your personal dos and don'ts. Let her find out slowly, if necessary. Save underwear with holes or obvious stains for when we're not around. If you stay for a weekend when you weren't expecting it, at least act as though it bothers you that you can't change your underwear, even if you couldn't care less.

 Upping Your Appeal

> As painful as it might be, ask a female friend to go through your wardrobe with you and tell you what works well, what's passable, and what needs to hit the trashcan fast.

The Truth About Penis Size

Just as we're concerned with the size of our breasts or shape of our legs, many of you worry about what we think of the size of your penis. You might poo-poo us for making far too much of various parts of our body, but we feel you do the same thing.

The Size of It

So does size really count? Many factors affect what we think of your penis. Yes, some women judge you and get turned on like crazy if you're well endowed. BUT, after discussing penises with many women (interesting conversations), I can say a good majority aren't as concerned about your size as you are. A large one may draw more ooh's and ah's, but a smaller one won't turn many of us off, unless you're totally inept at using it.

Some women are relieved if you're not too well endowed—a large penis can hurt. I've heard more complaints about lovers being too big than too small. A large one might be more visually stimulating but many of us find them painful. A long penis can hit the back wall of our vagina and hurt. More guys than you'd think say that having a very big penis is more a curse than a blessing—women get scared of it. Joe finds his a detriment:

> I have a very long dick—much longer than average. Women are scared of it. I don't fully enjoy intercourse anymore because I'm so paranoid I'll hurt my lover. After complaints from most girlfriends, I try not to thrust too hard or deep. It takes a lot of control when I'm turned on but I always worry I'll lose someone because I hurt her. So I have intercourse carefully, which isn't as much fun. Even when a partner asks me to go harder or deeper, I can't risk hurting her. So I'm on guard all the time. I hear men talk about how they'd like a big dick. Trust me, it's not the way women think. They may like looking at them but don't want them inside, or in their mouth. I wish I could shorten mine.

WHAT YOU HAVE IS WHAT THEY GET

Most women can be satisfied with organs of all sizes. You might need less skill during intercourse to satisfy her if your penis is thicker. Girth is what does it, not length. A thicker penis has the capacity to cover more area and is more likely to hit the clitoris. The bottom line is you can't change the size of your penis easily, so learn to work with it.

Relax, guys. A smaller penis can be compensated for if you learn how to use it! I once had a boyfriend who was very small. I admit, when I first saw his penis I thought "no way." I have news for you. He more than made up for his lack of size with thrusting moves that drove me crazy. I forgot his size quickly. The main nerve endings for stimulating us to orgasm aren't deep. If you learn to move your body well (see Chapter 14), you can give us as much pleasure as a stud in porno flicks, if not more. Does that make your feel better?

Macho Men versus Nice Guys

Many women find manly men sexy. But there's a difference between living up to the stereotype of being strong and protective, and living up to the stereotype of macho jerks attempting to prove their manhood, often with actions that are disrespectful/abusive to women.

MANLY VERSUS MACHO-JERK

Do you respect women? We're becoming more sensitive to men who don't show real respect. Some of you may have heard your father talking down to your mother. Men often did that when they handled financial needs and decision-making. You may not mean to talk condescendingly, but may come across that way—a habit worth breaking.

The macho mentality encourages some of you to talk down to women. Many of us get used to being talked down to just as you get used to speaking that way, but nothing justifies a disrespectful attitude. I warn women to be careful of guys with bad attitudes. If you don't get along with your mom, sister, an ex-girlfriend, etc., you may direct your anger or resentment at your current lady. We're all individuals. Holding on to a disrespectful attitude about women isn't fair to us or to you. It will ruin a relationship when she reaches her limit.

Keep the macho pressure in check when you're out with your partner. Don't act too differently with her around friends. If you usually hold hands, don't stop. Pay her at least some of the attention you normally would. We understand you might feel funny being too romantic in front of friends. But don't let macho attitudes break a good connection with your partner.

WHAT'S A NICE GUY?

A big complaint from you is "Why don't women give nice guys a chance?" There's a big difference between being a nice guy and a doormat. A nice guy is considerate, respectful, and honest with others and himself. A doormat tries too hard to please us, putting us before his own well-being or needs. A "nice guy"/doormat can be suffocating, always looking for how he can please us next. Too much!

People often try to please because they don't feel good about themselves. They hope that being extra special nice will make up for their perceived shortcomings. Don't feel bad if this is you. You're not alone! A large majority of men are insecure about at least something. This is normal, and you can work on any feelings of being less than worthy (more below). If you want to be attractive to women, work on your insecurities to lose the need to overplease. Trust me, when a guy is overly nice, we look harder to figure out why he's so insecure.

Self-proclaimed "nice guys" say they go out of their way to be nice to women and it doesn't work. Work? That means you're doing nice things for leverage. Wrong way to woo us! It tells us you don't feel good about yourself so you'll try buying us with kindness and attention. We read insecurity easily—it's unattractive. "Nice guys" are more responsibility. Let's face it. Many of you feel the same about nice women. If we're with someone who's bending over backwards to please, we feel pressure to reciprocate the kindness. Nice people are easier to trust but we may be afraid to trust. We like a challenge. But you can be nice without neglecting yourself. Marshall agreed:

> I used to complain bitterly about women dumping nice guys. I could never figure it out. There's nothing wrong with my looks but women rarely stayed long. They'd want to be friends with me because I was so nice. So I tried being a bastard. I got women but didn't like myself. Now I've brought the nice guy and bastard together for a reasonable mix. I still do nice things for a woman I'm seeing but restrain from doing too much. I do more for me. Now a woman I used to see who just wanted to be friends wants to date me again.

RECOMMENDATIONS FOR YOU NICE GUYS OUT THERE

You CAN be a nice guy who attracts lots of women, once you understand what nice really means. Nice guys can finish first, and get the best women! Here are things to keep in mind:

1. Be nice for the right reasons. I'm a recovering doormat. I consider myself a nice girl. I'm considerate of people's feelings and go out of my way to help folks more than most. BUT, I no longer put others before me. I'm nice because I feel blessed and enjoy being kind—not to keep people around like before. Being nice as a means to an end (making a woman want you) isn't nice. It's manipulative.

2. *Live up to the true definition of nice.* I love and appreciate true nice guys. They treat me with respect and consideration but show at least as much for themselves too. They're not self-sacrificing. They take care of themselves, have a strong sense of self, and enjoy being nice as I do. It took time to get a balance between being a nice door-mat and being self-centered. I tried the latter after my doormat days but didn't like it. Now I give to those I choose to and am respectful to everyone, even those who aren't nice.

3. *Don't try so hard!* Trying hard to please can be overbearing. We don't want to feel obligated to reciprocate excessive kindness. Don't do too much or try to impress us with gifts, especially early in dating. In a healthy relationship, we're attracted for who we are. I've had guys bring flowers on a first date. Wait until you know her better, although some women won't agree. We love getting flowers but it can be overwhelming at first. It takes time to identify how we feel. Flowers can put pressure on. We wouldn't give you a gift unless we really liked you so we may assume more importance from flowers than you intend. You may just be trying to get sex!

4. *Don't get fed up and join the ranks of bastards and jerks.* All you nice guys—please appreciate how wonderful being sincerely nice can be. Find a comfortable definition of nice and stay with it! The women you attract by not treating them nicely probably won't satisfy you in the long run and won't appreciate you. A middle ground can be found. Keep your sense of consideration and respect. Work on yourself (see the following section) to develop the balance needed to be a nice guy with a strong sense of self. Being nice should always include being nice to yourself.

Be the Nice Guy Women Want!	
DON'T	Do
Cater to her every need.	Ask her what she likes.
Always put her wishes first.	Treat her, and yourself, with respect.
Become what you think she wants.	Try to do some of what makes her happy.

Attractive Attitudes

The quality we find most attractive in you is confidence/self-assurance. Forget looks or perfect abs. To a degree, forget money. We love guys who think well of themselves; who speak positively; who know who they are and like it. I'm not talking about egotism or arrogance. Lose that. A healthy consciousness about you as a worthy, attractive, and capable man rocks us. Presence is very attractive. Both sexes notice people with a partner who's much more attractive and wonder why. Sometimes it's because of money or great sex. More often the attraction is a confident attitude that makes you incredibly attractive. Unattractive guys often attract very good-looking women because of how they carry themselves.

Dealing with Insecurity

Many of you don't feel good about something—too skinny—too hairy—potbelly—not enough hair, etc. Self-consciousness can make you hesitant to get undressed in front of a lover. If a woman puts your body down, do you want to be with that kind of person? If someone cares, imperfections are small in the bigger picture of who you are. *Never* point out your shortcomings. You may do it to get reassurance but we have eyes and can find faults on our own. Telling us is a turnoff. A guy actually told me on our first date that women always criticized him in bed. Forget sex with him! I didn't need to know that. Hey guys, confidence is *very* sexy so strut your stuff with pride.

Self-confidence transcends the details of your looks. I'm not body-perfect but walk proudly without clothes with a boyfriend. It's me, so he'd better accept it. It's you, so she'd better accept it. Guys are turned on by my attitude and comfort with my body and don't seem to notice flaws that used to glare at me. If you're uncomfortable with you, she'll pick up on it and scrutinize you more. Confidence helps focus on your good points. David was reminded in class:

> I almost forgot how insecure I used to be. Hearing some of you reminded me. Being 5'6" made me feel inferior most of my life. My hairline receded in my twenties and I thought I'd never find a woman. I dated but guess I always got in my own way. I tried too

hard to please to make up for my shortcomings. Nothing lasted. I'm a teacher. Ginnie worked at my school. We did projects together and got along well. I didn't feel insecure with her since we worked together. I assumed we'd be friends. One day, we decided to get something to eat and talked for hours. She said she enjoyed the time we spent. I couldn't believe it. We started dating and have been married for ten years. Without my insecurity showing, I was able to let her see the real me. Now I feel great. Ginnie loves me as I am.

Hair is a sore spot for some of you. Many of you are sensitive about it thinning. It lowers your self-esteem and confidence. If this is you, get a good haircut. Don't hide bald areas. It looks silly. Confident men let it show with pride. You've said women have commented about body hair—teasing if you have little or making a fuss if they think it's a lot. Some guys take care of too much body hair—they trim locks under their arms, around their genitals, and other patches of hair they're self-conscious about. Why not? Earlier I asked you to cut us some slack and not expect us to be perfect. How about cutting yourself some too?

DEVELOPING A POSITIVE SENSE OF SELF

In order to be as attractive as possible, work on how you view yourself. Confidence comes from good self-esteem. Here are ten steps you can take to feel better about yourself, which will lead to a more confident approach to women.

1. *Understand the true meaning of self-esteem.* Self-esteem means accepting yourself as you are, imperfections and all. My own definition is unconditional self-approval—being comfortable in your own skin. You can strive to be more than you are and have a lack of confidence—or be content with yourself as is.

2. *Accept yourself as a worthy person.* Self-esteem doesn't mean being happy with everything. It means accepting qualities you'd like changed. Self-esteem is your total picture as a person, as opposed to your accomplishments. See yourself as a person apart from your problems, without judging yourself by your faults. Being happy on the inside allows you more control over yourself in external situations.

3. Develop self-awareness. Start with a writing exercise. I never noticed my good qualities when I was focused on my shortcomings. I had to become conscious of my details to see past what I didn't like. List all the qualities about yourself that are positive—not just major accomplishments. Include having nice eyes, being friendly, having the ability to help others, making a great omelet, having good taste in ties, etc. Include what others praise you for. Add things you think of. Appreciate yourself because you have wonderful qualities. Stay focused on your good ones.

4. Cut yourself some slack. How do you treat yourself when you make mistakes? Do you beat yourself up? Forgive yourself and accept that you're human. Treat yourself as your best friend. What would you say to a friend who goofed? You'd probably reassure him. Stop using negative words, like stupid, to yourself. Learn to get past mistakes without putting yourself down! The way you treat yourself reflects on you. People treat you as you treat yourself!

5. Be kind to yourself by doing things that make you feel good. I treat myself every day. It can be simple, like giving myself permission to go for a walk, even when I'm very busy. I give myself gifts of love— a massage, delicious lotions, clothing I don't need but want, saving for a trip, tickets to see something fun and taking good care of my health with exercise, vitamins, and nutrition. I don't overdo spending but love giving myself a message that I'm worthy. When you do something special for you, no matter how small, it makes you more aware that you deserve good stuff. During a counseling session, Sal said, "Since I've done more for me I feel better and am noticing more confidence. Women respond to me better."

6. Show yourself love. Getting love starts with loving yourself. If you don't, why should someone else? Say "I approve of (or love) myself as is" often. While this may be foreign to you and hard to do, try saying it in a mirror. I enjoy saying "I love you." It eventually sinks in. Rob called a month after attending a class:

> I felt stupid saying "I approve of myself" in a mirror. It got easier. I can't believe I find it empowering now. I always focused on faults, like you said. I forced myself to write a list of my good qualities and was

surprised how long it got. It got fun adding dumb things like fixing my lawn mower. When I focused on faults, I didn't pay attention to my good features. Last week I took my son to a ball game and bought more expensive seats. It felt terrific. I'm worth it! My wife's seen a change and my self-esteem has even affected my confidence at work. I can't believe I'm saying this! I thought this was just for women.

7. *Nurture your faith.* Developing your spiritual side is a power tool. I had no faith until recently. Becoming spiritual meant developing faith in a higher power, which supports all aspects of my life. I learned to trust the Universe, then God, and felt the power. Find whatever higher being works for you. It doesn't have to be tied to a religion, though it can be. When you try it and see it works, trust intensifies. Faith keeps me whole, happy, and secure. When I'm not confident, I do affirmations to remember that everything works out fine. It always does. I began repeating "I trust in the Universe/God to take care of me." And I believe with all my heart that when the time is right—when you make yourself a healthy person—you'll meet someone. Until then, I enjoy my life instead of worrying about what's wrong with me.

Do You Have Appealing Confidence?	
AN ARROGANT/ SELF-ABSORBED GUY	A CONFIDENT GUY
Tells her what to do.	Asks for her input.
Looks at other women a lot.	Focuses on her.
Brags a lot—loudly.	Acts relaxed with who he is.
Blames mistakes on others.	Acknowledges his mistakes.
Knows it all.	Knows his limitations.

8. *Have faith that you'll attract the right partner.* I believe we attract what we put out. When you look enviously at your friend who's with a woman with her act together, realize he did something conscious or unconscious to attract her. Embrace a spiritual belief in whatever way is comfortable to get a power tool like no other. Accept that when you're ready, you'll meet someone healthy. Relax! Meanwhile, put your energy into creating a happy life that isn't dependent on a woman. That puts you into a win/win situation—you enjoy life with or without a woman.

9. Develop real confidence. Confidence is power. Few really own it, so those who do are attractive. When you have it, people want to be with you. But be aware that egotistical confidence can turn into arrogance, which limits the appeal. Women know that macho-confident men are probably putting it on because they're insecure. Exude confidence without being a jerk. Developing it requires facing and accepting you. It doesn't mean being tough.

10. *Fake it till you believe it.* Insecure people act insecure and come across that way. If we act terrific, we come across as terrific, even if we don't quite feel it. Force yourself to appear confident even if you're scared inside. Look her straight in the eye. Speak decisively. Work on your self-esteem to maintain your image. Eventually, the facade of confidence turns real. Jimmy said in a counseling session:

> *I forced myself to fake it and am starting to believe. Isn't that something? When we first spoke I was unsure of myself. I still am but not as much. I got advice on my appearance. Before I go out I say in the mirror "I approve of myself as is." That took time. It gives me . . . not confidence, but confidence to fake it, if that makes sense. I think more about what I like in me. Women think I'm okay now. I think I'm okay. I take on the role of a confident character and am an actor with women. But I'm becoming the character.*

What Women Are Attracted To

Do you believe that all we care about is money? It's absolutely not true. Unless you don't mind believing we want you for your wallet, focus on developing what you can. Download the information in this book for a better chance. Treat us with respect. Make an effort to communicate. Be thoughtful and romantic. No matter what you look like, you can incorporate these tools into your hard drive. Develop confidence first. That's your calling card. Then the rest can be implemented.

MAKE US FEEL GOOD

We love men who make us feel good about ourselves. I've dated guys who noticed every little thing that wasn't perfect and those who saw nice little things. I prefer the latter. Pointing out faults makes us self-conscious. When a guy notices the good in me, I like him more. Don't go overboard with compliments. A smile says a lot. A loving gesture and kind word go far. If you respect our opinions and show appreciation for who we are, many of us will want to keep you!

Don't talk about yourself too much. Show her that you're not a stereotypical self-absorbed guy by asking her questions. She'll feel good if you show interest in what she likes and thinks. We like guys who make us feel good. Say her name when you speak to her. It establishes and maintains a personal connection. She'll love hearing you say her name. Just don't overdo it. Go easy on using lines. They can turn women off. Some will fall for them so I won't say they absolutely don't work. Some women enjoy hearing those they want to believe. The best line is the truth. If there's nothing truthful to say, ask yourself why you're with her. Truthful lines should come easily if you like her.

KEEP OUR IMPORTANCE EQUAL

While confidence is attractive, getting too full of yourself or acting as though only your thoughts are worth talking about is a turn-off. Ask her questions. Don't trivialize what she says if you think what's going on in your life is more important. If it's important to her, respect that. Joe shared his experience in a group:

> I've been with Felicia a year. She talks about things I've found mean-ingless—what she read in a decorating magazine or what happened to a friend. Sometimes she'd cry if I didn't listen. Last week you said I'm marrying her for a reason. Even if what she says isn't important to me, it is to her. You said the best way to share a life is to respect her world. Felicia loves decorating—I've seen it as silly woman's stuff. You showed me that's unfair. It's not up to me what's important to her. I asked her why she enjoys some of the things I ignored before and find them more interesting now that I'm listening with an open

mind. It's part of Felicia and I can't push it away like it doesn't exist if we share a life.

Some of you talk about yourselves nonstop. Are you nervous or trying to impress us? If it's a macho thing, get over it or you'll turn us off if a conversation is always you. We might think you're a jerk if you don't leave room for interaction. Not giving her time to speak says you don't value her thoughts or feelings. Let her know how wonderful you are without words. Trust her to notice.

Make Yourself More Delicious to Her
Be a gentleman.
Compliment her.
Smile and make eye contact.
Be direct—with confidence.

What Women Want Most from Men
I asked women what they want. Here are their top answers:

1. *A man with an ability to laugh.* A sense of humor ranked high. Asia said, "I love a man with humor. He's usually easier to get along with. It makes working out problems easier." I want a guy I can laugh with, even in bed! But don't make fun of your partner. Some of you can be mean under the guise of humor. That's called picking on us—not funny!

2. Someone who can lighten up. We like men who are playful, with creativity and a desire to explore life. Don't be afraid to try new things. It makes you more interesting. The ability to let go and have fun is very attractive.

3. A man with a good balance between work and play. Workaholics aren't fun. I know because I've been one, which motivated me to develop my own concept for a balance, which many have adopted, called F & M.™ It stands for "Fun and Money." I get interesting reactions when I tell people I'm into F & M! I keep Post-It Notes saying "F & M" around my apartment to remind me I need a balance. Money with fun is definitely better!

4. *A man who treats his partner well.* Honesty, understanding, romance, compassion, respect, and loyalty were qualities most women emphasized as important in a partner. Also included as must-haves were lots of sex (smiling now?), reliability, courtesy, communication, and comfort. Adria said, "Treat me with dignity, respect, trust." Amy said, "I want someone who has utter respect for me and my feelings . . . an honest, supportive, and ambitious man."

5. *A man who is decisive.* While you shouldn't control us, approach us with ideas about things to do and ask for our input. We hate when you arrive saying, "I'll do whatever you want." Many of us hate making decisions and end up throwing "whatever you want" back at you. Ask what we like to do but have a backup. We like you to take charge while taking what we'd like into consideration.

Initial Meetings

There's no right way to approach us. What may turn one of us on can turn another off. It's best to be yourself. Would you prefer I give you a clever pitch? The bottom line is—a woman should want you as you basically are. You can *fake it till you believe it* to garner the confidence to approach her. But while a totally phony facade may get you laid, it won't create a foundation for something real.

★ | ### Make a Good Impression

If she's coming to your place, especially the first time, tidy up, make your bed with fresh sheets, hide photos of other women you dated, and have a scented candle handy.

We like being approached with confidence. If you see a woman you'd like to talk to, say "hi" and see if there's a vibe. You should be able to gauge her response. Is she friendly, polite, or encouraging? Initiate a conversation. Is she unresponsive or cool? You know what to do—move on.

Start casually. Find out her interests and suggest doing an activity together. Watch for lectures, events, or activities she may enjoy. Proceed slow. It's not easy to segue friendship into more, but try a little bit at a time. Or you can be honest and say you're attracted to her.

9

ROMANCE SOFTWARE:
REAPING THE REWARDS OF BEING DELICIOUS

S he's someone special and you like her a lot. You call when you say you will, which is something you haven't always done. You treat her as well as you know how, taking her to nice restaurants and picking up the tab. You think you're doing well, so it hits hard when she complains that you must not like her since you're not romantic. You were thinking you were. What does she want? ~

What Is Romance?

I looked up the word *romance* in several dictionaries. Most definitions referred to a fictitious love story. That may account for our different programs about romance. I said earlier that women have unrealistic expectations of you because of what we see in the media. We can go way over the top in our desire to recreate the romance we see in movies and read about in books. You may feel it's dumb to have to give us the romance we ask for. The bottom line is, indulging us with some of what we crave may please us so much that you're pleased too!

 Romantic Tip

Greet her on her birthday with a cupcake that has one lit candle. Extra points for singing "Happy Birthday."

We complain you're not romantic enough and you don't give us what we want. Yet we may not be specific about what it is. Part of our concept of romance is that you have a desire to spontaneously be romantic. We expect you to figure it out like the heroes in movies or books. This chapter has tools for satisfying our need for romance more easily.

I asked women to described what romance means to them. Here's a sample:

Julie: Being swept away. Thoughtful gestures and being genuinely considerate.

Mary: Time spent that is exclusively the two of you. Locking eyes, private jokes, etc. Spontaneity. Outward, unselfish appreciation for the other person. Creativity, sensuality, and letting your guard down. Secrets just between you two.

Diane: Getting to know me well and doing things based on a personal knowledge of what I'd like. Regular, simple, intimate gestures, like a quick caress or knowing eye contact. Affection. Knowing he wants to have contact with me.

Lea: Time spent because you want to—not because if you're sweet you'll get laid.

Adria: Little things here and there for no special reason.

Yvonne: Taking the initiative to make things special.

Judy: Thoughtfulness, attention to details, special treats.

Jenna: When a man shows he knows me. Personal touches—not just flowers.

Nora: Noticing my appreciation of something and following up on it—buying me something I've admired. Learning about a topic I'm interested in.

Amy: Thoughtful acts, giving of self, kissing, hugging, touching affectionately.

Vi: Spontaneous affection and gentle touches. A kiss for no reason.

Being More Romantic Without Getting Nauseated

Do some of our needs seem unnecessary or silly? Many of you said when you did something to show how romantic you could be, you were put down for it. Our expectations can get ridiculous. But if you're serious about pleasing us, romance is an area where you can get the most bang for your effort!

Think about how we show our feelings for you—kisses, affection, verbal expression, doing special things. We let you know how much we care in ways we'd like to be shown. We shower you with the kind of attention we'd like to get from you. We remember the occasions we wish you'd remember and fuss over. Admit it. Although we may do more than necessary, it feels good when we make you feel special. That's what we want from you—to feel special. Gestures that solidify our connection to you and say that you want to connect to us accomplish that.

It's the Little Things That Count—Again

Paula said she considers her guy romantic if he knows little things she likes. "Not materialistic per say. Just small things." The little things I spoke of earlier that create connections with your lady and show you care can mean the most. Jeff recommends, "Go the extra mile to show you care. The littlest detail makes a difference." Sam said, "Give her little surprises, thoughtfulness." Al advises, "Spontaneous gestures of affection."

A common desire that came across in what women said is doing things that are personal. We like to know that you pay attention to our preferences and take the time to please us in a way you think we'd appreciate. Greg says, "Find ways to make her feel special with small gifts showing you know what she likes. Give her regular affection, especially when she's not expecting it." Once a boyfriend bought me gold hoop earrings for my birthday. It told me he just bought something without thinking. Why? I only wear silver jewelry and had never worn hoops. Pay attention to what your partner likes. If necessary, get help from someone in finding something that shows you know her. Had my boyfriend bought me something smaller, less expensive, but that showed he'd paid attention and was trying to please me, I'd have been ecstatic. Gifts that are personal are more romantic than flowers.

Romance can be practical gestures too. Cut out an article that may be of interest to her. Bring her batteries if she keeps forgetting to buy them. Take the time to share knowledge about something that means a lot to you. Shirley said, "Rich made me feel very special when he took the time to explain some of the finer points of what he does as a geologist. It's his passion and now it interests me."

Romantic gestures say that we're on your mind. Romance is a symbol of caring. We want you to demonstrate your feelings and be considerate of ours. Get to know your partner to figure out what she'd appreciate most. Giving flowers is obvious and works on most of us. We know they're a no-brainer, but love them. Gestures that show you thought about what would make us happy mean even more. There are easy little things that can give us romantic gratification:

+ *Leave notes for her.* They can say "I love you," "Can't wait to see you later," "I had a wonderful time," "Hello," etc. Find a way to tell her she's desirable or you love her.

+ *Plan an evening to pamper her.* Play soft music, light candles, and offer a massage. Bathe her, wash her hair.

+ *Give spontaneous affection.* An unexpected kiss, tender caress, or hug once in a while can keep romance simmering.

+ *Say something that shows you appreciate a specific aspect of who she is.* Flatter her about something you really appreciate. It means a lot to me when a guy expresses appreciation for my passion about my work or the way I get something done. Noticing something special about her shows you're paying attention.

+ *Create a romantic date.* Make dinner by candlelight or take her out somewhere special. We love holding hands, cuddling, tenderness, and compliments. A firm or tender squeeze or brushing our arm with eye contact in public is romantic. Several women said their guy put rose petals on their bodies and made love to them. That's more work but the results rock!

+ *Telephone to just say "hi" or to say goodnight after a date.*
  Hearing from you can be romantic, especially when it isn't
  for a practical reason.

If you regularly use the suggestions you're comfortable with,
you'll get fewer complaints. Romance is an offshoot of the "attention"
we crave. Try some of the things from the beginning of Chapter 2
that create connections. Allow yourself to enjoy the pleasures you
share with her. Get into hugs. Don't just go through the motions.
Try losing yourself in a long hug. That's a connection worth making!

SPECIAL OCCASIONS

Don't forget birthdays and anniversaries. They may seem trivial
but mean a lot. If you're "not good at doing them" as many of you
told me, don't use that as an excuse or cut an attitude that they're
not important. If it's important to her, respect her needs. We take
your not remembering or caring about an occasion personally. If you
forget a date she holds special, she may assume she doesn't mean as
much to you. If you don't remember your anniversary, how special
can she be? Even if you think making occasions important is dumb,
acknowledging them makes her happy. It symbolizes caring. We're
happy with even small gestures that translate to caring. Say "happy
anniversary" first. If it's accompanied by affection or a gift, even better. Remembering is the important thing!

Romantic Tip

Say "happy anniversary" first—even if you set your alarm to wake
up earlier or say it after midnight the night before. A token (one
rose, a heart lollipop, diamonds) with it gets more mileage.

If you're bad at remembering occasions, ask your partner for
help. It may not be the most romantic thing but if she reminds you
a week before, you can remember. Ask for a list of special dates and
don't lose it. Write it on your work calendar but don't tell her. Ask
for ideas for gifts for appropriate occasions. Most women love jewelry or something personal. We like knowing you chose a gift we'd

like, instead of just copping out with flowers or something easy. If we mean enough, it's worth the effort. Not only will you have less complaining by remembering a special day, the look of joy on your partner's face should make it worthwhile. With just a little planning, you can satisfy what may seem like big needs.

Perfecting Your Kiss

A kiss can be the most important tool for getting what you want from us. Many women will bend over backward, tolerate stuff that we wouldn't normally, get in the mood for sex, and be more amenable to requests if you knock us out with a kiss. A good kiss is your power tool. It can set a great tone for a potential relationship and warms many of us more than you'd imagine. It can win us over or set a sensual tone for later. The most consistent response I got from women when I asked what they want from you on many levels was good kissing.

WHAT CONSTITUTES A GOOD KISS?

Good kissing isn't just putting your lips on someone else's and letting nature take over. Women often complain that they feel mushed instead of kissed. We like feeling special during a kiss. Ellen complained:

> Some men kiss like there's just one of us. Those types make me feel like I don't count—like the kiss is for them only. I've had men kiss me in ways that turned me off, yet when I tried telling them, they didn't want to hear me. I've tried subtly guiding them, and even blatantly asking them to switch gears. Most of them don't get it. A man who turns me off with his kiss will NEVER get further than that. A kiss is a barometer of things to come.

Some of you can be dense when you kiss and refuse to change course. You may think you know it all, or aren't concerned with our pleasure. Of course you're entitled to enjoy a kiss, too, as well as kiss how you like. But since you usually control a kiss at the onset, compromising on what we like gets you further. Plus, I'd bet anything that you'll like it, too! Every man I've guided through a kiss has come up breathless. Make her feel that way too! Use some of my suggestions to accomplish this.

We know a lot from a kiss—if you're passionate, warm, considerate, uptight, selfish, or probably a lousy lover. A big complaint from women is bad breath. Brush your teeth (and tongue) or use mouthwash before a date. They also hate slobbering wet kisses, too much teeth, sucking our mouths like a vacuum, too much tongue too soon. Mary elaborated, "I get turned off by a guy who's lashing his tongue around like it's some sort of workout or performance."

You don't want to be one we discuss as a kiss from hell. I haven't had many, but one guy was an example of being in your own world during a kiss. After our first date, he kissed me good night. It was gentle, tender, and light—a taste of something that could be sweet. He took me home after our second date and no sooner did we sit on my couch, than Mr. Kiss From Hell plunged his tongue deep into my mouth with no warning, tenderness, or initial contact with my lips. I wasn't even expecting a kiss and was stunned and repulsed. I tried pushing his tongue back with mine. As I tried extricating myself, he went to town. I gagged on what felt like a big, fat, wet monster. He was oblivious to my discomfort.

Some of you may be wondering what was so terrible about Mr. KFH's moves. Using your tongue is intimate and many of us need to get to know you. That was our first real kiss and he didn't allow passion to build by starting slowly. The worst part was Mr. KFH was out of touch with me. My reaction to his kiss was disgust. While he enjoyed himself, I was trying to pull away without hurting his feelings. When he came up for air he asked, "Wasn't that wonderful?" He assumed because he was loving it, I was too. That was our last kiss.

Don't be self-absorbed while kissing. Just because you enjoy it, she may not. Don't assume anything if she's silent. She may not be able to breathe! Start slowly, letting it build in small increments. Pay careful attention to her response. A kiss can instantly set a tone for later intimacy. Many women say that if a guy can't kiss well, he'll probably be a bad lover—less incentive for intimacy! Kisses that connect open doors! One that leaves a bad impression closes them quickly. Jessica explained:

I can tell a lot from a kiss. I love kissing—most women do. But we like to sense his feelings in a kiss. I've been with men with kisses so sweet I wanted to jump their bones. I've also been kissed by men who made me want to puke! Some slobber or use their tongue too soon. They don't understand how to work to brilliance. Yes, a kiss can be brilliant. I don't understand why all men don't kiss reasonably well. If they'd pay attention to what they're doing and our response—follow our lead sometimes and SLOW DOWN! It often feels like they're kissing to get us into bed, instead of as an act in itself.

Ally added:

I love tenderness. Soft kisses put me away—after I'm involved with a guy I adore the deep passionate ones do too. But not always at the beginning! When I don't know a guy well, I need to get used to him through kissing. If he jumps into a heavy kiss too soon, it puts me off. If I'm not comfortable, I can lose interest. I've been with guys whose looks were only borderline attractive to me, but when they kissed me tenderly, my interest increased.

GETTING TO FIRST BASE

Kissing is an art. Most men I've kissed say I'm a great kisser. I want to be and so I pay attention to it. I love kissing and now it comes naturally. My partner reads my feelings through my kiss. Yet many of you are stuck and may not even know it if no one felt comfortable enough to tell you.

Good kissing isn't synonymous with skill or experience, though you can learn to be good. Most of us appreciate if you start a kiss tenderly and build as we relax and get into it. Let your feelings or attraction for us motivate you. A great kisser gets in touch with his passion or attraction, and expresses it through nonverbal use of his lips. Think of it that way instead of as just physical contact. You shouldn't act! Tap into your passion. Dahlia elaborated:

Men can be boorish about kissing. Sometimes I feel violated from it. When I'm kissed for the first time and his tongue goes way into my mouth, I'm thinking, "yuk!" Of course there are times when chemistry is so intense that kissing can heat up and speed up quickly. But a man's taking a chance if he rushes a kiss. If I want to go faster, he'll know by how I kiss back. Men should pay more attention. Showing consideration goes a long way.

The First Kiss	
DON'T	DO
Use your tongue.	Gently brush her lips with yours.
Dive into her mouth.	Tell her you care.
Unleash your passion.	Gently caress her cheek with your fingers.
Go indefinitely.	Make eye contact as you approach her.

Practice. It may sound silly but kiss your own hand gently to see how it feels. Try different ways and experience the sensation each one creates. Then you can get an idea of how your lips feel. Get in touch with the movements, timing, rhythm, and nuances of a kiss. Are you thinking that creating the perfect kiss can be phony? When you see results, you'll appreciate it. Kissing is like dancing. You can go for years thinking you can't dance, stepping on toes, and feeling clumsy. Then you take lessons, go through awkward stages of practicing until you master it, and eventually feel as if you've been dancing forever. Kissing can be like that. Learn what feels good to us, practice, and it will come naturally in time.

TIPS FOR BEING A GREAT KISSER

Kissing may come naturally to some but you can all learn to be great kissers. A first kiss is important. Once in a relationship, you can ask what she likes and not be so concerned. But you have to get beyond the first kiss. Here are some techniques to make her want your kisses again. Learn the art and keep us happy!

1. *Start off slowly.* It's easier to pay attention to our reactions.

2. *Practice the art of kissing lightly.* It's a great opening to passion later. Make your lips feel like a feather as they touch her lips and face. Linger, almost in slow motion as you softly kiss. It will leave her wanting more. Kiss her face lightly. We love tenderness and often equate it with caring. Show you care by being tender. She'll tingle with romance.

3. *Use your hands gently to caress her.* A finger lightly across her face can relax her. Gently push the hair off her face. Cup her face in your hands—keep them off other body parts in the beginning. Don't turn us off by moving too fast!

4. *Keep your tongue in check.* Some of us like it immediately. More don't. Eventually, try the tip of your tongue on her lips to see her response. If there's no resistance, slowly enter her mouth. Try rolling your tongue around after kissing softly. Ideally, the tongue action should feel natural. Many of us love it after we get to know you.

5. Build slowly. As you feel her respond, press a little harder and add more passion and tongue. You should be able to tell if she's enjoying it. Too many of you act as if you don't want to know. Let the passion build up as you get to know her better or if she lets you know it's okay.

6. Make your first kiss count! It sets the tone for future intimacy. Prolong it as much as you can. Practice doing it in slow motion. Nibble her lower lip and then go back to tender. Once you have the moves, integrate your feelings with the actions. Don't fake it. Darryl said, "If there's no affection in a relationship, the kiss isn't there. It's just sex."

Let warm feelings you have for your lady inspire you! Get into the yummy mood that a slow, sensual, tender kiss can create. The more you kiss before sex, the more receptive she'll be. Don't be a robot, stiffly going through moves. Once you get a slow and sensual rhythm, relax and enjoy the results it brings! When she's with a guy she's into, Mary said she loves to be kissed:

> *Intense and passionate. Also little lazy kisses are fun and good for your soul. Strong, urgent kisses can be great. The mood should dictate*

*the style of kiss. Slow, deliberate good-night kisses are nice. What-
ever reveals feelings and passion, that's what a kiss should be about.
Be true to your instincts and attentive to your partner.*

Being Patient About Sex

You ask why we slow down your moves. We want a relationship and
value the importance of getting to know each other slowly. Courtship
is loads of fun. Building up sexual tension makes sex sweeter when
you're both ready. Lots of things can enhance a relationship besides sex.

BEING FRIENDS WITH YOUR LOVER

Often we're anxious for romance/intimacy and ignore friendship. We're human, so it's easy to fall for someone we're attracted
to, skip the preliminaries, and get to the sweet stuff. A meaningful friendship between a man and woman creates a solid foundation.
Developing a strong bond sustains support during rough spots.

Friendship is worth developing. We can fall in love with someone we don't totally like as a person and get carried away by good
looks, great sex, a need for companionship, or other attractions. Too
late we find ourselves living with or married to someone we don't like
or respect. Gabe appreciated learning this:

> *I used to fall for a woman and jump in. It was always wonderful at
> first. Then it wasn't. It's horrible waking up with someone you real-
> ize you don't know. I'd leave if I didn't like her as a person. It seems
> obvious to date someone you like and respect but when lust is high,
> it's easy to get carried away. When I met Karen we did things we
> both enjoyed. I wasn't even sure if we were dating at first but it was
> fun. We got to know each other slowly through our interests. By the
> time we made love our friendship was solid—it took us to another level!
> We can talk. This is the best—having my partner be my best friend.*

The more time you take to get to know a potential partner and
the longer you wait for intimacy, the more developed the friendship
side can be. If you date a woman with long-term potential, get to know
her before whisking her into bed or melting her with romance. Get

small tastes before going for a meal. I know how desirable it is to jump her bones if you're attracted to her. But sex changes the nature of a relationship. She might want more from you. You might get scared and want to pull back. The dessert of desire may prevent you from thinking clearly about what kind of person she is. Waiting makes the end sweeter. One of the most delicious things I can imagine is falling in love with someone you like as a person too. Things fall into place easier when friendship is there already.

Romantic Tip

Mail her a note inviting her to a nice dinner. Ask her to dress up. Even if you live together, leave and return with flowers.

ROMANCING TO INTIMACY

"I Want a Man with a Slow Hand." The Pointer Sisters made that song a major hit, and it became the theme song for many women, myself included. This isn't just for the bedroom. Handling us with slow care in almost every aspect of dating and beyond will be gratefully appreciated by most of us. The gentle caresses you give at the beginning, without pushing for more, helps us relax for future intimacy. Cementing intimacy out of bed before going further creates a wonderful foundation of trust that makes sex the best. Many of you said you love the intimacy sex creates when it's with someone you care for. Those of you who haven't developed an appreciation for this, try it. Intimacy is delicious for both sexes!

Caring words and compliments represent romance to many of us. Expressions of feelings and appreciation can make us want to go the distance for you. I'm absolutely not advocating deception on any level of a relationship. I recommend always saying what you sincerely feel. But if you have nice thoughts about her, say them. We can get turned on in our heads before getting physically aroused. Saying the "right words" can get us started: Sweet compliments. Expressions of what she means to you. Reminiscing about fond memories between you. Telling her what she loves to hear is one of the best ways to put her in a good mood. Remember, we need reassurance. Words give that to us.

10   REDEFINING NAUGHTY: ENJOYING A SEXUAL WOMAN

Your girlfriend enters the room wearing a raincoat. As her buttons open, you're treated to a view of her in just a garter belt and stockings. She slithers out of the coat, slowly unbuttons your shirt, and does a seduction number on you right out of a porno movie. This has been your fantasy for years. You revel in the pleasure of her moves. But the next day you begin to wonder if you really know this woman you've always thought of as sweet and nice. The next time you see her you pull back and are hesitant to make love again. "Why do I feel this way?" you ask yourself. "Isn't this what I wanted?" You have no answer. ~

Isn't it wonderful to have a girlfriend who makes erotic moves on you? Or do you wonder what kind of woman she really is and how many other men she's done this to? Do you question or walk away from a woman who has sex with you from the beginning? Can you handle a very sensual girlfriend who likes to take the initiative? Or are these scenarios better left for your fantasies?

Rushing into Sex

"Don't women believe that men are more enlightened about sexual women?" is a question men ask a lot. NO! We know many of you aren't, though you'd like to think you are. Sexual stereotypes stay with both sexes. You say you want a sexually open woman but may run quickly if you get one.

We're all programmed to expect women to be ladylike. A sexual one doesn't fit that program, no matter how it turns you on.

WHEN IS IT TIME FOR SEX?

Many of you say you'd sleep with an attractive woman as soon as she'd let you. Warning: if there's potential for a relationship, wait until you know her well. Sex creates intimacy that you may not be ready for. It's hard going back to casual after crossing the line. Expectations are created. Physical intimacy can drive you apart if one of you gets scared or tries changing the nature of your relationship. Alex warned, "Men don't learn. They push and push for sex right away and then it doesn't work out. I don't try so soon anymore."

The heat of passion, or alcohol, can push us into bed too soon. If you want sex with someone you like right away, can you handle it without bolting? We usually expect more commitment. You have a reputation for panicking if you get in too soon. Fear of commitment and getting hurt comes into play since we usually take sex more seriously than you. Be careful. She will expect more after sex.

STEREOTYPES ABOUT EARLY SEX

I asked men after how many dates it would be okay for a woman to have sex and not have you think she's a slut. The average answer was after three to five dates. Alex added, "Men respect a woman more who says no." Yet many of you said you'd sleep with us as soon as we'd let you. I've never heard a woman judge a guy who had sex early. We don't label *you* sluts. So why do it to us? Joe shared in a group:

> I'm guilty of this double standard. I met a lovely woman at a seminar and had coffee after. She spent the following day with me. We had a wonderful afternoon at the park and dinner. She felt very right. I was excited when she asked me in. We kissed and got turned on. I wanted to make love to her—she said it was too soon. We kissed and I pushed for sex. Her resistance weakened after I told her how well we clicked and it seemed natural to continue. I assured her I wouldn't think badly of her. But I did. I'm ashamed but I had thoughts about her being too easy. Was she a slut? It was wrong but

everything I'd heard friends say about women who had sex easily haunted me. I stopped seeing this lovely woman and hurt her. I wish I could change this belief. Why was it okay for me and not for her?

Guys share beliefs and expectations, just as we do. They're part of our programs and are reinforced by our friends. Some of you discuss sex when you're with the guys. If you hear often enough that a woman is a slut if she doesn't wait through a proper number of dates, you believe it. It's not your fault but it's still egregiously unfair—one of the worst double standards. Be honest—why is it fine for you to sleep with us quickly when it's not fine for us?

★ **Important!**

After the first time having sex, contact her within twenty-four hours. We wait anxiously to hear from you, to know you're not judging us as easy, or running scared, or you just wanted sex.

Conflicting Desires

We're supposed to be sexually enlightened and own our sexuality, right? Wrong! Dave said, "I think a lot of women have the same urges but don't show them for fear of becoming stereotyped." Many of you are torn between your need for a relationship with a "nice girl" and your desire for hot sex with an uninhibited woman who rocks your world. What's a nice girl to do if you question whether both can be found in one woman? Society says it's okay for you to have a past, but not us. Do you really prefer less than great sex?

Approach/Avoidance to Sexual Women

You fantasize about us taking the initiative. You dream of women who talk dirty, wear a garter belt and stockings, and know how to get it on in bed. You wish for one who knows what she wants and asserts her needs. Okay. Here's the reality. Many of you say you can't handle this in a woman you're involved with on an emotional level.

Although it's the twenty-first century, many of you still suffer from the old Madonna/whore syndrome. Ideally, you want a sexual partner. But, you also want a partner who's sweet and innocent. Madonna/whore = "nice girl"/sexual girl. It's hard for many of you to see a sexual woman as nice too, which is a crock when you think about it! Just because we're enthusiastic about sex, doesn't mean we sleep around or have more experience than you. We sexual women can be self-conscious and stifle our sexuality for fear of scaring you. Most of you said you'd love to be with a sexual woman, BUT many had reservations. You acknowledge they're unfair but have them anyway. Here's a sample of common concerns.

> **Vernon:** I hate saying it, but when a woman is very sexual I wonder about her. How many men has she been with? Is it me who's turning her on or just having sex?

Why does enjoying sex mean we had a colorful past? A large majority of very sexual women don't enjoy sex with just anyone. We're more selective than many of you said you were. Just because many of you sleep around when you're horny, doesn't mean we do.

> **Gary:** When I'm with a very sexual woman I wonder if I can please her.

Hello! We wouldn't be having sex with you if we didn't like it. Being into sex doesn't mean we expect acrobatics or special techniques. Don't let your fragile ego keep you from getting involved with a sexual woman. We're naughty but still nice!

> **Clyde:** I like a woman who makes me feel like I'm the best lover she's had. How can I bring her to new levels if she's probably been to them already?

I was very inexperienced with my second lover but every pore of me responded to him. He assumed I'd been around many blocks. After getting to know me, he apologized for that assumption. But I was less responsive with my next guy because some men assume that a woman who enjoys sex is very experienced. They unfairly want to see responsiveness build over time so they can take credit for it. If you're making her moan—she enjoys you as a lover. Don't read beyond that!

Demetrius: I wouldn't want a woman to act too sexual—then I feel like an instrument.

That's how we feel. If both of you enjoy it, why feel used? Appreciate us if we're into both you and your penis! Most women wouldn't be into your penis if they weren't into you first.

Rob: The more sexual a woman is, the more I'm reminded that there were men before me.

Get over needing to delude yourselves that she was virginal until you. Don't ask how many partners she had. Leave the past in the past. Unless you can claim to have no history, accept that she's got one too.

 Romantic Tip

Personalize sex by using the word you. Instead of "Sex feels good." say "I love being inside you." Or "You amaze me." Focus on her, instead of the act. She'll feel more connected.

Give us a break, guys! Stop reading things into our sexuality. Get to know us before sex. Develop trust first so you have less reason to question our morals. Do you feel threatened by wondering if your partner is experienced? Do you question how many men she has had? Are you afraid she'll expect higher standards? Lose those doubts. Sexual doesn't mean an inordinate amount of partners or being loose. Leave the past alone. Brett told a class:

Joann is very sexual. When we first had sex, I wondered about her past. She seemed to know instinctively what I wanted and I never enjoyed a partner so much. I almost spoiled it by questioning her. I wanted to know how many guys she'd been with and if I measured up. But I didn't ask. I think highly of Joann and trust her judgment. I'm not one to judge. My past is quite colorful. I wouldn't like knowing Joann's was too but I have no right to hold her to different standards. We just got engaged and she said that one thing she loved about me was I didn't question her past. Her last boyfriend assumed her sexual nature meant promiscuity, which wasn't the case. She'd done nothing she was ashamed of but felt no good comes of comparing ex-lovers. She's right. I still don't know her past and don't care anymore. What's important is what we have now.

When we love sex, you may feel obligated to get it up for us, instead of just having sex at your will. Do you feel pressure to achieve? Some of you can be controlling and may want to control our sexuality too. If we make moves, you feel like you're losing it. Hey, sex isn't about control! It's the quality of the connection between us and the satisfaction we each get from it. Please re-evaluate any concern about satisfying a sexual woman. Don't take it personally if we suggest trying something different. Lighten up and enjoy! Arnold told a class:

> *I used to be uncomfortable with a sexual woman. I worried I'd never please her. If she took the initiative I'd doubt my ability or feel less of a man. Suzie changed me. She loved sex but let me know she loved sex with me. I felt comfortable enough to ask for guidance and got lots of it. She emphasized there was nothing wrong with me—she just wanted me to know what made her body respond. After Suzie, I found myself attracted to sexual women. I am planning to marry my very hot girlfriend. Sexual women are happier to guide you. Then you become a great lover!*

Too many of us repress desires because we're scared to let you see them. We deny our sexuality so we don't lose our "nice girl" status. If you continually put out even subtle messages that there's a double standard between your sexuality and ours, you'll continue to program us to stifle ourselves with you and save our wild natures for our partners that run on batteries. Am I making myself clear? Why miss great sex because of old programs? Ian said he likes a sexual woman. "There's less searching for boundaries and more getting to the fun, satisfaction, and experimentation you really want. Yeah!"

Nice Girls Can Be Horny and Love Sex

Many of you love the combination of "good girl" and "bad girl." It's not your fault if it intimidates you too. That's part of your program.

Sexual women and nice ones are rarely the same character in movies and on TV. A sexual woman is often portrayed as a bad girl. "Nice girls" aren't portrayed as sexual. Some of you find sexual women desirable, but not to have a relationship with. Eva told a group:

> I've been intimate with three men. My first didn't like virginity. I was insecure about being a good lover. It was great with my second. He was patient and I became sexual. Now I'm with Tom. We have great sex but he's uncomfortable with my passion and love of sex. He questioned my enthusiasm, not believing I've only had two lovers. I felt cheesy. He recently acknowledged he's seen my body response change and now believes I wasn't experienced. Should I be relieved or angry? Why can't men accept our sexuality at face value? I thought he'd be thrilled with a sexual girlfriend.

Nice girls have the same sex organs. Why can't we use them freely? Many of us love sex for the physical gratification, but we've been taught it's unladylike to enjoy sex too much. Get this—it's not just okay for us to love sex and be as horny as you. It's as normal, healthy, terrific, and as needed by many of us as it is for you. I love sex but I'm not a slut! I'm a very nice girl, yet self-conscious about my sexuality at times. Get used to us sexual women because we're here to stay! Be patient. Ron agreed in class and advised the guys:

> Get to know women better as friends. When you talk to them on that level, you may be surprised at how many women you think well of are very sexual. I started out talking to my sister. I honestly wasn't expecting her to smile so much when she told me how much she enjoyed sex. It helped me to see that it's normal for women to be into sex. Hearing other women talking about their feelings has been enlightening. Now I'm seeing a sexual woman. In the past I'd have been too concerned to relax. Now I'm loving it!

Helping Your Partner "Loosen Up"

As open as I am today, it took patience and caring on the part of several boyfriends for me to get comfortable with my sexuality. Many of us need "permission" to feel free in bed so that it doesn't take away from our being "nice girls." Many of us already know it's okay but want to know you're not judging us by our sexual response.

Self-Consciousness About Sexuality

Julie said, "Boyfriends have called me 'oversexed.'" When *you* crave sex you're real men. When women crave sex we're judged. Carmen said, "I love sex but most boyfriends act like I'm a nympho. I do nothing more than they do. Now I'm self-conscious about sexuality." Add to this our general programming to be insecure about our bodies. Insecurity inhibits us sexually. If we don't feel good about ourselves, exposing what we see as our unattractive body makes us uptight. Our self-esteem can be even lower in bed. If we're self-conscious, we may not be able to relax during sex and will want the lights out. Larry told me in a counseling session:

> I was married to Arlene for fifteen years. During that time I rarely saw her naked. She'd put on her nightgown first and then remove her underclothes when we got ready for bed. She reversed the process in the morning. Now that we're divorced, I look back and feel sorry for her. Wish I'd understood more back then to reassure her. I had no idea what to do and felt I must have been doing something wrong. I wish I had encouraged her more.

Some of us worry about how you feel about our genitals. As kids we may have been taught it's dirty "down there." When you touch that area, especially during oral sex, we're self-conscious. Your genitals are held in higher esteem than ours. Terms like "family jewels" and other macho phrases describe yours. What do we have? Pussy? Bush? Clinical terms like vagina? Many of us don't have the loving relationship with our genitals that you have with yours. Susan said:

> My mother said it wasn't nice to touch myself. I had to wash my vagina carefully or the smell might offend someone. It's impossible to not have some odor and I always felt dirty. Friends don't talk about this—I had no one to ask what was normal. My body image was awful. I'm attractive but was afraid a boyfriend would get turned off

if he discovered my body wasn't perfect or thought I smelled funny. I couldn't open up during sex until my husband said he loved looking at my body naked and my odor turned him on. Bless him!

We need reassurance in bed—to know you find our naked body attractive and that you enjoy touching our private areas—to know our natural odors don't offend you. Keep your nose away if it bothers you. We can't control what happens to our bodies. Many of you say our natural scent (this word is so much nicer—more sexy than *odor* or *smell*) is an aphrodisiac to you. Those of you who don't enjoy it— loosen up a bit. This is the scent of your woman and can be enjoyed. Our scent gets stronger when we're aroused, which should arouse you more. Help us be less self-conscious about our bodies.

COMMUNICATION IN BED

Why does our communication go cold when you try heating us up? Many of us are uncomfortable discussing sex. Even if you ask what we need, many of us don't know, or can't tell you. We may also be ashamed to say what we like. If you ask, "How do you want me to touch you?" we may not answer (more in Chapter 11).

Encourage her to open up. Give her permission to be sexual! Help her learn about her body. Gently let her know how you like being touched. We're used to you putting us in the mood. Say you'd like her to be more adventurous, initiate sex, and try new things. Tell her your needs and be patient. It takes time to undo the messages that said nice girls aren't sexual. Lauryn said:

I've always enjoyed sex but never knew what was going on. I'd lie back and enjoy what was done, some more, some less. If a boyfriend asked what I liked, I'd say "everything"—I didn't know. My husband insisted we talk about sex. I almost died—I didn't want him to know how ignorant I was. He made love slowly and tried different things, asking how they felt. I learned what got me going the most. We tried things together and I was honest with him. His love, consideration, and patience allowed me to open up. Our sex life has improved dramatically. Now I say more, pay attention to what I like, and take the initiative sometimes, all because he made me so comfortable about talking to him.

 Sexy Tip

Ask her to be the boss in bed. You'll only do what she tells you to. Keep it light at first—like a game—to relax her. Start by having her direct you to remove her clothing.

SUPPORTING OUR SEXUALITY

Appreciate our efforts at being sexy. Don't put us down for spending a lot of money on a piece of lingerie since you'll "be taking it off anyway." Wearing something we like makes us more comfortable with how we look. Until we're comfortable with our bodies in front of you, it's hard for some of us to indulge in wearing things like garter belts. Some of us may try it if you're patient and supportive. Many of us don't know how to let go and be a sexpot. Your expectations can be so varied that we don't know what to do. If you help us relax enough to get into the pleasures of sexuality, we may slowly allow our instincts to take over our sensibilities and put us over the edge.

We see a big difference between having sex and making love; sex and romance; horniness and passion. We attach too much emotion and meaning to sex. We expect too much beyond physical gratification. We want the trappings: intimacy, kissing, tenderness, snuggling, soft words, attention, feeling we mean something to you. You may want these too but also want physical relief. I warn women that you often think with the wrong head. I'm not criticizing you for it. You're entitled to your sexuality. But we do sometimes get misled when you're horny and momentarily give us the trappings to get satisfaction. Be merciful!

We need permission to be adventurous. Find ways to let her know you'd enjoy her being more assertive. We're torn between programs that nice girls aren't sexual, fear of you judging if we take a risk, and desire to let loose and tear you apart in bed. You have the power to redefine our "nice girl" program, to reassure and encourage us in exploring and experimenting with sexuality, and to bring out the sexuality we're all capable of experiencing with you. Positive encouragement can work wonders! Patience, sweethearts!

Sexual Fantasies

We all have fantasies. Some would be construed as more "normal" than others. You've asked if it's okay to try living out fantasies. It depends on what they are and who you're with. Many fantasies are better left to daydreams. If your partner is open, share slowly. Couples say they enjoy *discussing* fantasies during sex more than actually *living* them. If both partners are cool with it, try one for real. Living out any fantasy starts with developing a strong sense of trust. Go slowly and be sensitive to her response. Establish in advance that if either of you gets uncomfortable, you'll stop immediately. John told me:

> It took time to tell Jeannie about my fantasies. She was shy and I wasn't sure how she'd take them. I got a book on fantasies and asked to read some aloud. It led us to each tell one of our own. Jeannie liked how it turned me on and got turned on too. We both liked the idea of making believe I picked her up in a bar. We tried it one night. She got dressed up and went to a bar. I acted like I didn't know her. We flirted, I picked her up and seduced her. We had great sex and do variations once in a while. Most of our fantasies are just for talking about but this one's harmless and fun to role-play.

I recommend Nancy Friday's books on sexual fantasies. They've helped many women understand we're normal when we get sexual thoughts, erotic desires, and a need to masturbate and have multiple orgasms. Couples say that reading the fantasies in her books out loud turned them on. If your partner is uptight, encourage her to read one. Knowing other women have sexual feelings can help her relax and enjoy. Seeing that others have felt guilty can alleviate her own demons. It can also help your partner see that you're not as perverted as she may think when you share a sexual fantasy.

Pornographic movies turn on many of us, but first we need to be comfortable with you. Many women assume if you like porn, she's not doing it for you or you're not attracted to her. Some of us feel self-conscious about our bodies if we see perfect ones on film and know you're turned on. Keep your connection with her strong. Let her know that she ultimately is who turns you on. Some of us may feel threatened and nothing can reassure us. If you read porn magazines and she objects, I suggest having a talk with her rather than reading on the sneak. Explain why you enjoy reading them, that it's a pastime, and that it has nothing to do with anything she's lacking. This is another compassion spot. Help her relax with her sexuality and you may create new fantasies that she wants to participate in.

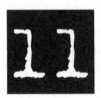

Is She Having an Orgasm?: The Dynamics of Female Sexuality

Sex has been great between you and your girlfriend. She acts like she enjoys everything you do to her. You look lovingly into her eyes. Your face is excited, expectant, and eager to hear a positive answer as you ask her, "Did you come?" All of a sudden she doesn't look happy anymore. She says you ruined it for her. What's wrong? Don't you have a right to know if you've done your job properly? Shouldn't you be informed if she *has an orgasm?* Why *do some women get so uptight when you ask them?* ~

What's Wrong with Asking, "Did You Come?"

If you ask, "Did you come?" and you're looking at us expecting to hear "yes," what do you think we'll say? We know if we say "no" we'll burst your excitement and your ego, so many of us say "yes" whether we did or not. When you're waiting for the answer you want to hear, we don't want to ruin the mood with honesty. Think honestly about what you'd like to hear at that moment, "yes" or the truth.

Female Performance Anxiety

Reaching orgasm is harder for most of us than it is for you. Our genitals aren't right out there like yours are. More of our ability to come is in our heads. While a mental turn-on enhances your sexual feelings, physical stimulation does the trick. Our bodies don't always work that way. Our state of mind has the ability to open us up or shut us down. We can be on the brink of an orgasm and lose it instantly if there's a distraction, like an inquiry.

In the past, only you got performance anxiety. You still worry about getting an erection and keeping it up. Women also get performance anxiety—about having an orgasm. We use mental stimulation to build one and anything can be an orgasm buster. The phone can ring and break our reverie. Feeling you getting tired of stimulating us creates pressure to come. We're more likely to fake an orgasm, since we can't push our bodies to get off quickly. We don't work like that.

The worst orgasm buster for many of us is four little words. Asking "Are you almost there?" can stop an orgasm in its tracks. As your orgasm approaches, do you want to give a progress report? When you're lost in a blowjob, do you like us asking how long you'll be? Since our ability to have orgasms is more fragile than yours is, asking affects us more. We lose ourselves in the sensations and joy of your touch. As we get closer, we focus on feelings going through our body. But we can lose it in seconds if you ask about it. "Are you almost there?" is like sticking a pin in a balloon. It deflates many of us quickly. Laura said:

> Jake's the best lover I've had. He doesn't have super skills or lasting power but is considerate of my needs. When I met him, I'd given up on orgasms with men. I was focused on faking them and never relaxed to actually have one. Other guys said they wouldn't be satisfied until knowing I'd climaxed so I didn't come, I performed. They'd be pleased with my performance and stop. Jake started out asking me what I enjoyed. He let me know he wanted me to feel good. What a switch. He never asked about orgasms. I stopped faking and allowed my body to enjoy him. This man allowed me to come by not putting on pressure. Sometimes I do, sometimes I don't. He knows the truth and is fine with it. He wants me to be satisfied in whatever way works for me. What a sensational lover!

Sexy Tip

Stop focusing on just getting to the orgasm. Slow down and pay attention to every sensation along the way. Let her response to your touch turn you on more.

Whose Orgasm Is It Anyway?

Do you want to know we're satisfied, or do you want to know you gave us an orgasm? Think about it. Many of you assume that for us to enjoy sex, we have to have one, so you ask for confirmation. Some of you sincerely want to make sure we're satisfied. But some of you want to hear "yes" no matter what the truth is. If you need to know, ask yourself why. For your ego? As a confirmation of your prowess? Your need for achievement makes our orgasm a goal for some of you. Our satisfaction may be a distant second. Women complain some of you don't listen. Your quest for an orgasm can be more important than what we'd like. Wanting to give us an orgasm for you, not for us, doesn't please us. Janelle complained:

> Earl keeps asking if I had an orgasm. I've asked what's his problem but he just says he wants to know. "Why?" I ask. I could be on the brink of an orgasm and this man breaks it by opening his mouth. "Did you come?" I feel like a game in a carnival and he's trying to get rings around something to win the prize. My orgasm seems to be the prize. This man beams when I say "yes." If he'd shut up more, I'd mean it more. But I don't think he cares. Men and their egos!

Those of us who are easily orgasmic are thrilled if you want to make us come. But many of us are prevented from having one when we feel pressure. Ask your partner how she feels and go from there. If we want to have one for you we may try too hard. See how she feels. Make sex more fun and less goal oriented!

Faking Orgasms

Many of us don't ever fake orgasms because we have them easily. But more than you might think do fake, at least sometimes. We'd rather have real ones but aren't secure enough to make you go the distance. We don't want to fake but have no choice. Give us what we need—not what you decide we need—so we can both be satisfied.

The Pressure of Your Messages

Many of you are very considerate about pleasing us and I thank you for that! Most of you who don't quite get it are running on your original program that allows macho to seep into your need for us to come. You give us subtle, or not so subtle pressure to have an orgasm. More than a few of you indicated that if we did a good job of faking, so be it. When I asked, "How important to your pleasure is it if we have an orgasm?" well over 50 percent of you said *very*. I asked why it's so important. Let's talk about some of those reasons:

> **Sam:** Men are supposed to give women orgasms. They complain we don't care about it so I work very hard to make sure my partner has one. I expect her to tell me when she does.

It's a wonder some of you don't ask for a written report on how you did. Sex is supposed to be fun. Ask her what she wants!

> **Craig:** Giving her an orgasm makes me feel like a man. Guys say they do it all the time so I should be able to, right?

Wrong! Our orgasm isn't a bull's eye on a target. We're women, not one of the games you and your friends play to see who gets the highest score. Your friends may all be with women who fake. A real man finds out what his partner wants and gives it. Please detach your egos from our orgasms!

> **Jon:** I get very turned on when she seems to be coming. It enhances my pleasure greatly.

What about our pleasure? This attitude reinforces that we need to come for you, not us. Our arousal should turn you on and our being satisfied should be good enough. If you get turned on by acting, hire an actress or watch a porn film!

> **Gregory:** I'm left hanging if I don't have an orgasm during sex. I can't imagine a woman being satisfied without one.

Stop trying to imagine and listen. MANY OF US CAN BE VERY SATISFIED WITHOUT AN ORGASM! If we tell you sex was satisfying without one, it usually was. You don't know our bodies better than we do. Accept what we say. If we lie, it's our responsibility if we're not satisfied. Respect our choices.

Glenn: It's more fun when she comes too! It feels more mutual. I don't feel right getting mine if she doesn't get hers. If I have an orgasm, shouldn't she have one too?

Reciprocation is admirable but our bodies can't come on your cues. Your pleasure shouldn't hinge on our orgasms. You may not be satisfied if you don't believe we're satisfied, when we are. What a silly waste of what should be good sex.

Judd: I feel like a failure if a lady I'm with doesn't come. Am I doing it wrong, or is something wrong with her? I've gotten angry if women admitted they didn't. If she was into me, wouldn't she get turned on enough to come?

No. Our orgasms involve more than that. Don't take them personally. Many of you say you do. You're only a failure if you ignore what we tell you.

Why We Fake

Our good girl program taught many of us to give you what you seem to want—our orgasm, even if we fake it. We sacrifice pleasure for security. Many of us need more stimulation than we think you're willing to give. The pressure of you working hard to bring us to orgasm makes us too self-conscious. Here are reasons women fake:

Susan: I take it personally when I can't have an orgasm: I worry if something's wrong with me. Men do that by asking in accusing ways why I didn't come. Then I wonder what's wrong with me—I love sex and feel satisfied. Men say all women have orgasms. They make me feel guilty so I fake.

Maybe all their women faked! We can't help our bodies being different. There's nothing wrong with either of you if she doesn't come easily. Because we don't understand our bodies well, many of us think not reaching orgasm is our fault. You can take away our pleasure by making us feel inadequate.

Louella: I feel stupid if I don't have one. I've had partners make such a big deal out of the orgasm that I was afraid of losing them if they knew I didn't have one. Sex is supposed to be pleasurable yet I'm so uptight about orgasms that it's not. I rarely have them so I fake. Then men are happier with me.

Judith: I'm afraid my boyfriend will leave me. I hate disappointing him.

We feel like failures if we don't achieve for you. Some of you said you'd consider ending a relationship if she didn't have orgasms with you. Women say this has happened. Our having an orgasm is so important to some of you that you won't stay if we don't always have them. So we perfect a fake one.

Kendra: When I first had sex with my beau, he was insecure so I faked to give him confidence. I need more stimulation for a real one but can't tell him after faking so much. He thinks he's a stud and I'm an idiot for putting his ego first.

Peni: I may need more time than I'm comfortable asking for. Eventually I fake an orgasm to put my boyfriend out of his misery. I wish I could get him to go the distance but he makes me feel I take longer than most women.

Many of us worry that if we ask you to keep giving us stimulation, you'll be annoyed. Our good girl program makes us uncomfortable asking you to go the distance. We take longer than you do. Learn to enjoy bringing her there if you don't already. Let her know you do.

LaTonia: I usually have orgasms with my man. At times I know I won't no matter what. I may be tired or my body just doesn't want one. I'm satisfied without one but my man will go all night if he knows I didn't come. So eventually I fake. Maybe he'd understand if I told the truth but others haven't. Sometimes I can't handle more stimulation.

Stephanie: Sometimes my boyfriend tries too hard. If I know it won't happen for real, I fake to give him a break. He doesn't believe that nothing is wrong between us if I don't.

Barb: When I've had enough and my guy would take it personally if I don't come, I fake.

Sometimes our bodies don't orgasm, just because. Even women who have regular ones say they're sometimes satisfied with sex but can't come. We can't explain it and worry you'll think something is wrong, which usually isn't true. Relax if we don't always have an orgasm. Don't take it personally!

 Sexy Tip

> Before sex, kiss her tenderly—then stop and gently stroke her body. Then kiss with more passion. Stop again. Keep building until she's relaxed. The more you kiss, the more responsive she'll be later.

How We Fake Orgasms

Many of you said you can always tell if we come but more said you can't. Some of you said you don't care if we fake since it turns you on. Can you tell? When I saw the movie *When Harry Met Sally* with my boyfriend at the time, he laughed. He couldn't believe we could fake orgasms like Meg Ryan. You should have seen his face when I broke into some authentic sounding moans and serious orgasmic noises.

How do you know if she really responds? Do you feel our muscles twitch? We can fake noises and muscles contracting, we can arch our backs, but we can't fake wetness. If we get wetter and wetter, we're responding. Some of us get wetter than others. Not being wet doesn't mean we're not aroused or didn't come. But wet doesn't mean orgasm. We can soak ourselves just from being aroused. That's fine. It means we're enjoying sex. Be happy about that!

About Our Sexuality

You'd be shocked if you heard how many women attending my seminars ask what an orgasm feels like because they're not sure they ever had one. Hello! That means they didn't. Others can have them on their own, but not with you. I want to explain how our bodies work with our minds so you know what you're up against.

OUR MINDS, OUR BODIES

As I said earlier, we're not brought up to like our body or to be comfortable with it. Sexuality is exalted in men. It's not that way with us. We don't have nice terms for our genitals. What can we use if we even want to talk about our whatjamacallit!?

A big difference between us is that you own your sexuality. We don't. Your body signals arousal via erections. Our signs are subtler—we often miss or don't recognize them. Since we don't discover sexuality easily, we may not have learned. Early programs tie sex and love. Some of us don't know we're supposed to get excited. Dee didn't learn until adulthood:

> When I was a girl, I had no idea what sexual feelings were. I knew boys masturbated but my friends and I laughed at it. I thought my vagina was something my husband would put his penis in for his fun and to have a baby. At sixteen, a boyfriend put his hand in my panties. He asked if it felt good. I didn't know it was supposed to! He was shocked. I was embarrassed. It took two years until my body woke up and I enjoyed a boyfriend's stimulation and even more years before I masturbated. My boyfriend can't believe it. But how could I learn if no one talked about sex? Guys get hard-ons. When I'd feel funny down there I thought I had to pee. All my mother said was that I should wash thoroughly down there or my smell would offend people. My friends never discussed it, except to laugh at boys. There were no books, no one to ask. We're brought up with such guilt that most of us would never touch ourselves, even if we felt tingly. It's a wonder I ever learned.

Many of us discovered sexuality later than you, if at all, and expect you to open ours by pushing the right buttons. We put a burden on you but often can't give directions. Why do you think many of us have no answer, or say "everything," when you ask what we like? We may not know! You guys have it easy. Your genitals are up front. You get comfortable with your penis since you handle it often. It's a friend, a source of self-pleasuring, the core of manhood, your pride. Many of you said you learned to stroke it young, often by accident. You don't have to look for it. It's easy to reach out and touch.

Our hot spots aren't as easy to find. We have few accidental orgasms, and don't know what they are if we do. Most of us don't make friends with our genitals as girls. Very lucky ones learn early. Lucky ones learn early in adulthood. A large percentage of us take a long time, or never find our pleasure points. Many of us grew up seeing our vaginal area as an unattractive, smelly place. Some of you reinforce that. We're taught to be clean. Period. So why touch it? Our clits aren't an obvious place to put our fingers. Many of us don't know what a clit is until you find it!

Some of us never have orgasms. We haven't explored our sexuality and no one showed us. It's not simple for us. If we rub your penis, you'll probably come. We can't always find our clits any easier than you can! That's right—many of us are unfamiliar with our own bodies. David shared his experience:

> When I began having sex with Joyce, I asked what she liked. I got the pat "Everything." I said I wasn't a pro but wanted to please her. She confessed she didn't know. I asked if she knew where her clit was and what it looked like. When she said "No" I asked for a mirror so we could explore together. We laughed as we searched for her clit and examined it. She said she'd never had any source for learning about her body and was shy. She's happy I made her look. It gave me a chance to know her body better. Now she knows it better too. We're getting good at communicating what turns each other on.

If we never had a patient lover take time to please us, we may never have learned to open up sexually. Help us find our way! If you want the best chance for giving her an orgasm, get to know her before going for yours. If she gives evasive answers, try different things and ask what feels best. Explore us. Lead us. Monica told a class:

> When I lost my virginity, my guy had no idea—he did a slam-bam thing. My next guy asked what to do. I didn't know. I can't blame men if we can't guide them. But they need to understand our ignorance. Some of my friends are in the dark about their bodies too. If men don't take time and help, they'll never please many of us. My husband gave me the greatest gift. Eric wanted to give me pleasure

and proved it. He tried all sorts of stimulation until I responded. As I relaxed, his patience continued. When I had my first orgasm, it was a team effort. Now we have the hottest, most intense sex possible, all because my husband gave me a chance to trust him enough to open up.

A big factor in having an orgasm is trust. Many of us can't let go because we're scared of what our bodies may do during an orgasm and worry you'll get turned off. Will we pee or get too wet? Or let out gas? Will you be turned off? The moment of an orgasm is a loss of control. We need to be comfortable to let go. Let us know our scent isn't a turnoff—that you accept us as we are—that you enjoy looking at our body—that you're not in a hurry and will stimulate as long as it takes. Help us relax so we can share our sexuality. You'll love it!

Masturbation

You ask how much we masturbate. Many of you think we all do. But many women say they don't masturbate regularly, if at all. It's hard for us to talk about it. We gab about almost anything to our girlfriends, telling every detail of our sex life (sorry—it's true) but we rarely speak of touching ourselves. If there's no one to tell us, we may not know we can masturbate, or how. That's why I included a chapter on masturbation in *All Men Are Jerks Until Proven Otherwise*. Many of us are enlightened about our bodies. Many aren't. Jaydie shared:

I didn't know women masturbated until I was twenty. Bob saw I didn't have orgasms and asked if I had them alone. I was horrified. Bob explained it's normal for women and gave me a vibrator. I was scared and confused but eventually it worked. As I learned about my sensuality, I talked to my best friend and we encouraged each other. Growing up I saw my vagina as taboo to touch, except to wash. I'd get aroused during sex but never understood it. Bob is history but I owe him my sexuality. I've educated friends about the joy of masturbating. I'm much more orgasmic with my husband because of it.

Some of you said you don't like knowing your partner masturbates. Your egos wonder why we need more than you give us. We may give ourselves orgasms more easily because we know instantly if we hit the right spot. Sex for one involves the same partner so practice makes perfect. While I can't speak for all women, I know that a large majority of us don't feel masturbation comes even close to being a substitute for making love to you. But it keeps us in tune with our sexuality. The more we do it, the hornier we get. Louis learned to appreciate that:

> *Elizabeth and I always have great sex. I never knew she masturbated until I walked in on her rubbing herself when she wasn't expecting me home. Had I known she did it, I'd have wondered why I wasn't enough for her. But I got so hard watching I couldn't believe it. By the time she saw me watching, I was working on myself. We both kept going and my orgasm almost knocked me over. I loved watching her techniques and use them on her. She said she's always enjoyed getting herself off. It gets her more excited for me. Now I love it. We sometimes masturbate together and then get it on together. It's a big turn-on.*

When you're in a comfortable relationship, see if she'll masturbate with you and do the same. It gives each of you a chance to see how the other likes being touched. Seeing how she brings herself to orgasm can help you become better at it. If she doesn't masturbate, encourage her to do so. Judy said:

> *Gary always asked what I liked in bed. I couldn't answer—I was ashamed admitting I'd never had an orgasm but enjoyed sex. When I finally told him, he went down on me for ages but I couldn't relax to come. I was scared of what would happen. Gary encouraged me to explore myself. I finally had an orgasm on my own. Once I got over my fear, I began having orgasms with Gary. I loved sex before. Now it's even more intense.*

Hot Tip

Watch an erotic video with her that's not porn—*Body Heat, 9½ Weeks, Henry & June*. Hold and caress her tenderly when you do.

The Dynamics of Pleasing Us

Too many of you complain that we take too long to come. You admitted impatience, getting tired, or wanting to have your orgasm and go to sleep. Many of you, God bless you, expressed joy and enthusiasm at the thought of stimulating us to satisfaction. But those of you who don't feel this way feed our hang-ups and self-consciousness about taking too long. Let her know you love pleasing her. Tell her how good it feels to taste or touch her most private parts.

Can we enjoy sex without an orgasm? Yes! Yes! Yes!! Get this, guys—our bodies operate differently. A large majority of us say the quality of the sexual experience determines our satisfaction—the sensuality, the passion, and the range of physical contact that satisfies us. Of course we'd like an orgasm too. I won't lie. But it's not nearly as important to us as it may be to you. Lisa said, "I'm more satisfied by intercourse without an orgasm than by giving myself ten." Although many women want one every time to be satisfied, many, many women feel the same way as Lisa.

If you want to satisfy your partner, ask what she needs when you're out of bed. Must she have an orgasm each time to be satisfied? Put more energy into making her feel good instead of into achieving orgasm. Instead of "Did you come?" ask questions like "Do you need more?" "Would you like me to keep going?" "Are you satisfied?" "What would you like me to do?" Make it seem like a pleasure, not a burden. Focus on just finding out if she's satisfied or if she'd like more stimulation. Orgasms will come!

Getting Past Issues

We all have issues that affect our sexuality. As you get older, you may not feel as virile, which can affect your interaction with women. Some women have a bad attitude about sex, for a variety of reasons and you might not know why. A surprisingly high percentage of women were sexually abused as children. Many were raped. Some women only had lovers who didn't care about their pleasure or who made them feel used during sex. A loving partner can help her heal her wounds and learn to relax and enjoy sex. These women often need the most patience.

Sexually Violated

It's hard for many women to relax and enjoy sex when negative memories are attached to it. If she hasn't disclosed anything and you suspect she was sexually violated in the past, wait until you've established lots of trust before trying to find out. When a woman is made to have sex against her will it becomes an act to avoid, not enjoy. Counseling is imperative for her to heal, but she may still have aversions to sex. If your partner has scars from sexual abuse, go very slow. Do what you can to earn her trust. Set boundaries so she's more comfortable knowing you won't go past her comfort zone. Women can learn to love sex, if you care enough to take it slow. Jody shared:

> My father and uncle both used me sexually from the time I was eight. My mother knew but ignored it. They forced their hands into my private places. I had to rub and suck them. As a young teen, they forced me to have intercourse. I didn't know who to turn to for help. When my first boyfriend made a move on me I screamed. Eventually I got married. My husband knew my history but was a slam-bam-thank you ma'am lover. I hated sex even more. When I left him, I avoided intimacy. My next few boyfriends tolerated my lack of response during sex. Jack didn't. He got me to talk about it. He didn't force sex and was very loving. Slowly he helped me to distinguish between sex with a man I loved and being raped. I now thoroughly enjoy it. Women like me need tremendous patience and understanding. Slow and loving can make the difference. Jack took the time to help me learn about my body and find out what aroused me.

Women who've been sexually abused have a lot of shame. Sheila said, "I felt like a piece of dirt after I'd been raped, unworthy of being loved. A voice keeps telling me I could have done something to stop it." One of my clients got no love at home. While visiting family at age five, her "uncles" took her to a room and played with her vagina. They asked her to lick their penises and do other things. Doreen said she liked it at the time. Their touch felt loving to a child who'd been starving for physical contact. They loved what she did to them—the first positive reinforcement she'd gotten from an adult, and they gave her candy after. This went on for two years. As Doreen got older and understood the truth, shame ripped at her. How could she like something so wrong? She's still struggling to get beyond it, and to relax during sex. John went the distance for his wife. He says it was worth it, explaining:

> *My wife was sexually abused. She went through the motions with me in bed but I knew she wasn't into it. It took a while till I got her to tell me how she felt and why. She wanted to enjoy sex but it reminded her of being raped in college. We focued on cuddling and caressing at first. It was hard not to push for more but I wanted her to want me, not just feel obligated. Eventually she trusted me more. I must emphasize it was a very loving time for both of us. While I was frustrated on one level, the intimacy that developed based solely on our feelings for each other was something I had never experienced. Slowly her guard went down and I was able to touch her in a sexual way. When she had her first orgasm, it was a very deep moment for both of us. Now she's been able to put her bad experience into persepctive and keep it out of our bed.*

GETTING OLDER

Getting older creates issues. Sex can be a little different as time passes, but still terrific! Jerry says, "Just because we're over fifty doesn't mean that a part of our lives is not longer available to us or wanted. Divorced and widowed people are missing out of one of the greatest times of their lives. The second life is just beginning after fifty and some of us need help in sorting out what to and how to behave in our new sexuality." You can have sensuality at any age! Just be aware that it can take a little longer to warm up and stay warm as you get older. It may be better than you expect. Edwin, age eighty, says:

> *My sex life is not affected as much as I used to wonder. I thought it would mostly be over and gone by seventy. I still have sex but not as often. It takes about a week to recover. However, there is no difference in the joy and the feelings of loving. The main thing about my erections is more fore-play is necessary. My partner also needs more to get ready. I never tried Viagra, and am a bit leery of it. But I have used injections, and they are okay. I think if it were not for my diabetes, I would need nothing.*

Eat bananas! The vitamin B in them increases the blood flow to the penis. There are many things both medical, such as Viagra, and organic, such as herbs for energy and blood circulation, that can help you get and maintain an erection. Regular cardio exercise helps keep the blood flowing everywhere. Get regular checkups and follow your doc's suggestions for staying healthy.

Some women are more difficult to deal with as they get older, if they still have low self-esteem. Aging makes us crankier. We feel even less attractive. Changes in our bodies can make us feel even worse. The older a woman gets before she enjoys her sexuality, the more ingrained her hang-ups become—unless she meets a very loving, patient man who helps her overcome the negatives she's experienced. But all these issues can be dealt with if you're with someone you care about. Menopause can cause a woman to lose her desire for sex but there are products to help that. Explore different products if she's open to them.

CREATING AN ORGASMIC MOOD

To maximize the potential for your partner having an orgasm, create a mood as relaxing as possible. Be patient. Act willing to wait for as long as it takes her to come. Slow and sensual sets the best conditions. Be romantic. Get her in the mood before you're in bed. Hold hands. Smile. Express your feelings, even if it irks your practical side. Let things happen naturally and stuff your ego away so you don't go at her body as though it's a task to conquer. Relax and enjoy. If you do, she's more likely to have an orgasm. Focus on what she says satisfies her and not on making an orgasm your goal.

Communicate with your partner. Be open to asking questions and letting her know you truly want to give her what she needs. Pay attention to what she says rather than doing what you please. If you listen to her obvious and subtler responses to your touch, you'll learn exactly what she loves. The longer you're with someone, the more easily you'll know how to hit the right buttons to satisfy her. Earn her trust with all of the above. The following chapters offer specific directions.

12 HEATING HER UP: HOW TO GET HER REVVED FOR SEX

You're with a woman you really like. The evening was romantic. You take her home and she asks you in. All systems say go for it. Her eyes invite you. You kiss her gently. She responds with enthusiasm. You tell her what a terrific evening it's been. She agrees. Your next kiss is more intense. She sighs. You caress her face and she's smiling. You caress her neck and shoulders and she's still smiling. As you shift your body on top of her and caress her breast and more, she jumps up and accuses you of just wanting her for sex. What did you do wrong? She was so into you.~

Do you want the hottest, most intense sex possible? Would you love your partner to look forward to being with you because you drive her wild in bed? The process starts in this chapter. You can have the most precise sexual techniques but they're not worth much if we're not receptive to them. Even those of us who love sex can be uptight about how you treat us. We want to feel you're with us for ourselves, not just to get laid. We need to be reasonably certain you want to make love to us in particular. We don't want to feel all your sweet tenderness and affection are just a means to get us into bed. All your good intentions to be a great lover can fail if you think you can bypass foreplay with most of us. She may go along with you but probably won't be satisfied or enthusiastic the next time.

When you minimize the importance of foreplay, you also minimize how much pleasure you'll get. An enthusiastic partner will rock your world in bed much more. Foreplay is the appetizer of sex—like the lubrication that makes your car run smoothly. An appetizer whets the appetite for a meal. Heavy-duty technology goes into a car but without simple lubrication, it freezes up. You can have sex without foreplay but why risk that her body isn't ready? Foreplay is easy, fun, and the best prelude for pleasing your woman in bed. A warmed up partner wants you! She'll be much more responsive to your touch and your needs.

I must emphasize that what's traditionally referred to as foreplay shouldn't just be a means to intercourse. Arousing all parts of our body constitutes sexual play. I think of intercourse as one facet of sex. Foreplay IS sex! It builds intimacy. Touching, caressing, knowing glances are all part of making love. All aspects of foreplay arouse us and are part of the act of sex. It prepares us for intercourse but also gives us orgasms and is satisfying on its own. Enjoy it all!

Condom Consciousness

Foreplay begins with safe sex. Women say many of you don't want condoms and do whatever you can to avoid them. This is a wake-up call, guys! I don't care how nice you or she is, or how carefully you choose a lover. You're at risk.

Why You Should Use a Condom

You hear warnings, yet many of you don blinders and try to talk us into skipping condoms. Stupidity rules when you're in heat. You give lame excuses for not using them. I don't care if you're drunk or out of condoms. Take a cold shower and wait! Forgive my lecturing but I've known too many "normal," educated, clean, heterosexual men who got AIDS and other sexually transmitted diseases (STDs) from "normal," educated, clean, heterosexual women. Yet you don't take it seriously. Gary explained:

> I hate using condoms! A condom takes pleasure away. Some women insist on them but I'll do anything to convince her not to. I have good judgment. The women I date aren't the disease kind. They're classy and well brought up. I can't imagine them having something. Just thinking about that possibility gives me the creeps!

Think and get the creeps! Men lie—women lie. Studies indicate that many people wait until a relationship is on solid ground before telling a partner about an STD. Some don't know they have a disease since not everyone has symptoms. You can't be sure, no matter how squeaky clean she seems. Sheila confessed:

> I have herpes. It grosses me out that I, a nice girl, could catch something. I got it from a boyfriend who never told me he had it. He thought as long as he wasn't having an outbreak I was safe. Well I wasn't. I left him but have to live with this for the rest of my life. It's a nightmare. Do I warn guys I sleep with? No. I suggest condoms but if they're too stupid to use them, what can I do? I hate arguing about it. I try being careful and have sex when I think I'm not contagious. But my ex did that and look what happened to me.

ARGUMENTS FOR NOT USING A CONDOM—DISPELLED

These days, you have as many excuses or rationales for not using condoms as there are condom varieties. Here are some common ones. Have you used any?

- ✦ **"Nice people don't get diseases."** AIDS and other STDs may hit some groups more than others, but "nice" people catch them too. Herpes and other STDs are as prevalent among educated professionals as in other groups. Don't assume that only certain types catch them. Be careful! Safe sex isn't about your ability to discern which women are safe.

- ✦ **"It doesn't feel as good with a rubber."** You complain the sensation during intercourse is lessened or it ruins pleasure completely. We don't like them either! Sex without a condom is definitely more pleasurable. But, isn't your life worth more than a great orgasm? Besides, there are many great condoms on the market that are thin enough for you to forget you're wearing one, if you allow yourself to. Men who've accepted condoms say it still feels great with one!

- ✦ **"Shouldn't I trust her if we're in a relationship?"** Safe sex has nothing to do with trust. Almost all my boyfriends said they trusted me enough to skip condoms. How can anyone know someone is disease free? If you care about each other, getting tested should be a step toward building trust in a relationship.

+ **"Condoms affect my erection."** You've said it's embarrassing when you can't get it up. You're nervous having sex for the first time. Condoms put more stress on your erection. You admit you've used condoms and kept an erection, but dwell on times you lost it. Get used to them! Let your partner practice putting it on you sensually. You can get used to condoms as a regular part of sex. Practice makes more perfect hard-ons while using a condom!

+ **"Thinking about catching a disease means thinking about the men in her past."** Be real. We all have a past. If you don't want to deal with it in the future, protect yourself now. Lenny confessed:

When I met Sara, I knew she was someone I could be with for a long time. She didn't push to use a condom and neither did I. I didn't want to consider someone like her could have a disease. Six months later I found myself infected with herpes. She confessed she knew she had it but thought we had sex during a safe time. Now I have it for the rest of my life. I didn't want to talk to her about past men. She seemed so sweet and innocent.

+ **"I use condoms until I get into a relationship."** Her past is still there, guys! STDs don't always show their ugly faces for a long time. Laura said, "Todd and I were careful at the beginning but when we moved in together four months later, we felt we could stop using condoms. I found out later I had vaginal warts and now we both have them. I'm so ashamed." Play it safe—get tested with your partner first.

Speak to a potential lover about safe sex before the heat of passion. Stopping safe sex after a relationship solidifies isn't safe. Get tested for HIV *and* other STDs—the only way to be confident. Get over excuses! Too many studies indicate a large percentage of you won't accept how common STDs are in ALL people. Ignorance is no excuse! Using condoms sometimes protects you sometimes! You may hate them but infected men say that's much worse.

 Sexy Tip

> For a more natural sensation, put a few drops of a lubricant (Like Body-glide by Eros) *inside* the condom at the very tip before putting it on. It provides a slippery feeling and helps you forget you're wearing one. Just make sure that the condom fits you snugly at the top so it doesn't slide off.

Make safe sex more fun. The resource list at the end of Chapter 15 has mail-order companies for condoms, lubricants, and HIV home-testing kits. Try different ones. Some condoms are thinner and more comfortable than others are. Call the Center for Disease Control National HIV and AIDS hotline at (800) 342-AIDS for places to get tested. Some do it free. You and your partner should also get tested for all STDs. We can't take chances!

Warming Her Up

You're turned on. She seems to be too. Your penis is throbbing as you grind against her. She pushes against you. You both undress passionately. Your southern head says go—you act on impulse, putting your penis into what seems like her welcoming vagina. It feels so good. When it's over, you're feeling wonderful and want to languish in that just-laid glow. Your reverie is ruined when she cuts an attitude, saying that you're selfish and were thinking only of your own pleasure.

Foreplay shows you take time to satisfy her. It says that making love to her is more than just having intercourse. You can be very satisfied from just screwing. Many of you incorrectly feel if you can come gloriously from intercourse alone, we should too. Our bodies don't work like yours. You heat up quickly. Many of us can't. Foreplay lets us heat up as you calm down a bit. It can bring you both to a more equal state of arousal. And, she will love you for it!

The Importance of Foreplay

Although we enjoy the physical aspects of sex, most of us are more dependent on mental stimulation. We don't just get a hard-on and feel ready to go. We need to be relaxed and feel you care. We want trust. Foreplay provides some of that. At first, it allows us to get used to being intimate with you. Foreplay gives us the romance and tenderness that loosens us up and gets our juices flowing.

Think of foreplay as anything that arouses, not something that needs to be done. It's not just stimulating our genitals or getting us ready to be entered. Foreplay can start with a simple connecting gesture. It can dance us through tender romance, and take us to the height of passion and arousal before genitals are touched. Foreplay isn't just for us. Once you expand your concepts, foreplay can bring you to a level of sexual pleasure you've never experienced before. The anticipation it creates can make sex an experience that brings you closer to your partner, intensify your pleasure, and make your partner so pleased that she'll go out of her way to thank you—with actions!

WORDS THAT AROUSE HER
"I love to hold you."

"You feel so good."

"I love your body."

"Sex with you is so special."

"Being with you is the best!"

"Seeing you naked makes me so hot."

"I'm in love."

THE SEDUCTION OF WORDS
Your well-chosen words can add to great foreplay. Words can be a turn-on for both sexes, but for different reasons. Most of you would like to hear, "You turn me on," "I'd love to screw you," or something with a sexual overtone that makes you feel manly. We're more into compliments, statements of feelings, and words of appreciation that are more personal and less sexual. Words create a connection. We want to know you want to make love because you like us, not just

because you're horny and we're handy. "I really love being with you" goes over better than "I'm hot for you." If you're in a long-term relationship, tell your partner that she still turns you on like crazy.

Hot, down and dirty, explicit sex talk absolutely has its place. Some of us like it right away while others may never allow it. A majority of us can accept/love it as part of sex play, once we're comfortable with you. We need to be comfortable with other parts of intimacy first; to trust your feelings; to be relatively sure that you won't get turned off if we talk dirty back. Discuss sex talk out of bed. Even if we say it's fine, test slowly. See how graphic you can get. Dirty talk turns many of us on too, when we're comfortable. You might want to tell your partner how much it arouses you when *she* talks dirty.

Satisfying Foreplay

The best kind of foreplay is given with the intention of making us feel good. Connecting with our emotions is much more important to most of us than having a lover with Olympic lovemaking skills. Tender caresses and the attention you pay to stimulating our genitals shows you want us to feel good. When we have that, we can relax and enjoy more.

WARMING HER UP

I recently drove a car that hadn't been used for weeks. Being in my usual hurry, I pulled out right away. It made scary noises. I parked and let it run for ten minutes to allow the fluids and oil to lubricate the car's engine, and then it ran properly. We're not cars, but warming us up is a similar principle. Taking time to heat us up in the beginning loosens us up and turns us on so our responsiveness to sex is maximized. Why enter a dry woman when you can enter a wet one? Why make us fake an orgasm when you can give us real ones?

It takes us time to warm up. You can ignite quickly. We simmer until we reach a boil. If you don't seem into continuing foreplay or you're just waiting for us to get off, we get self-conscious and say it's enough. Too many of you said you think women need too much foreplay. We know that and those of us still operating on our "good girl" program let you get away with not giving us enough. But it doesn't lead to great sex.

If you care about your partner, foreplay shouldn't be tedious. Think of sex as sharing pleasure instead of just give-and-take. You should enjoy foreplay too. Tell us what you like. Show us how you enjoy being touched. David said, "As a forty-one-year-old male, I need foreplay too!"

As I said earlier, foreplay is actually the wrong word for all the titillating, delicious turn-ons and "everything but the intercourse" stimulation. Sex doesn't have to always end with intercourse. Pretty much everything else is referred to as foreplay, yet it can be terrific, satisfying, and final play on its own. Foreplay pleasure can hold its own as sex. Don't sell it short by seeing it as a means to the good stuff. Done right, it is the good stuff!

SENSUALITY AND PASSION

Sensuality and passion are qualities that most of you love experiencing from us but don't allow yourselves to give unconditionally. Many of you are so in control that you can't completely let go during sex until orgasm. It's a delight to be with a guy who not only groans as he explodes, but purrs, smiles, and says how good it feels throughout sex. Your response turns us on. If you're subdued and we can't tell you're enjoying it, we worry. If you'd lighten up in bed and relax and enjoy it thoroughly, you'd get more pleasure. You all say a noisy response from us turns you on. Why deprive us of that pleasure?

When asked if you made noise during sex, a majority of you said a variety of Robert's "The 'usual' during the release." There's nothing "usual" about an orgasm! The stimulation and pleasure is there for the entire time. Sam said he's embarrassed to make noise. Do macho men not enjoy sex? Is it unmanly to let go? Believe me, plenty of you have learned the joys of vocally responding during sex and we praise these men. If my lover groans, I get more aroused. I never heard a woman laugh at it or think less of him. Au contraire—we think more! Try some oohs and ahs to get comfortable. Open up a little bit at a time.

Sensuality is appreciation for little nuances that enhance our womanhood; responding to touch, even in the supermarket, because we turn you on; feeling warm, tingly, and happy when feeling the deliciousness of soft fabric, a gentle hand, a soft kiss, a caress in the shower, etc.; understanding why I refer to so much as "delicious"! Getting lost in pleasure and allowing yourself to express it is sensual. Andy said, "I feel I shouldn't make noise during sex." Later he said women complain he's not passionate. Hello! When will more of you embrace the very essence of sheer joy, a total appreciation of life's treasures and pleasures flowing through your body, enveloping your being—PASSION!

What exactly is passion? It has many definitions, but to me it's the aphrodisiac of life. It turns on my senses and heightens my awareness to the joys of seeing and doing and feeling and tasting and touching life's experiences. Passion is a deep, soulful, warm, and intense feeling of enthusiasm for whatever touches me. It's unconditional living and feeling, surrendering control of joy to unlimited heights. Passion is very attractive to others. It shows a zest for living, and ignites passion in those you come into contact with. Get in touch with your passion and ignite your partner! Let loose in bed. Taste slowly and let it build. Surrender to desire and pleasure during sex. Let enthusiasm and appreciation take you over during sex. As Madonna said, "Express yourself!" The rewards are great.

 Hot Tip

Suggest taking turns reading aloud together from a sexy book. Look for those by Susie Bright or Nancy Friday for starters.

The Many Aspects of Foreplay

Foreplay is anything that gets you or your partner aroused. It stimulates your desire for sexual activity on many different levels. You can have foreplay any time, any place, anywhere, even when you're not together—over the phone, with notes, e-mails, by fantasizing about suggestions you give each other. There are many levels of foreplay on my sexual menu. I will be making an analogy to food because many of you say you find food sensual. Enjoy these delicious treats!

FOREPLAY SNACKS

Before dinner we can get hungry for something tasty that whets our appetite. You can indulge in foreplay snacks when you're not home or if others are around. They keep you and your partner focused on what will happen later. Following are things you both can do to heat up earlier in the day so anticipation can drive you both a little (or a lot) crazy (some of these are better with a long-term partner or someone with whom you know you're on the same sexual wavelength):

+ Call her at work and say or allude to what you'd like to do later. It can make it hard to sit still at work but anticipation can make for hot sex at night.

+ Create a signal for use in public. If one of you uses it the other knows you want sex and can't wait for later. It can be a thumb's up, scratching your nose, a tug on their hair—any creative sign you make up. It's fun to get aroused secretly.

+ Give her casual intimate touches in public. Besides holding hands, use fingers to gently caress her. Touch various parts of her arm when speaking. If you're sitting next to each other, lightly touch her shoulder or tickle the back of her neck or head. All these things increase the intimacy we desire.

+ In a restaurant, feed each other, licking food off fingers or lips sensually (within the bounds of good taste for public behavior).

+ Read poetry to each other at home, in the park, over the phone. It can put you into a delightfully sensual mood. Then you can write your own!

+ Wear a cologne you know she likes. Ask her to help you choose one. A sexy cologne can turn some of us on like crazy!

+ When you're in public, flirt with her. Tease her with winks, intimate signals, licking your lips, a pinch, hug, or kiss. See her as the sexy woman she is and let it show in your attitude and subtle actions toward her.

FOREPLAY HORS D'OEUVRES

What I call foreplay hors d'oeuvres get us relaxed and into a sexy mood. We can be uptight, tired, or just not into sex and may not respond to sexual overtures. But the right words, caresses, kisses, and other romantic canapés can heat us up quickly. Following are things women recommended to relax us into a mood for hotter activities. These may not seem like foreplay since they're not overtly sexual. But if they heat her up, does it matter? Try them and you'll probably have a partner who'll go to the ends of the bed for you:

+ Lightly run your finger over her body, drawing make-believe pictures and writing your name on her skin. Give a gentle pinch now and then.

+ Kiss her face gently all over. Slowly put a tender kiss on each closed eyelid, her cheeks, forehead, ears, etc. Save the lips for last and savor each drop as your mouth finally settles in on hers and the kiss gets deeper and deeper.

+ When you kiss, look deeply into her eyes for a connection. Let her see your desire for her. Let her feel your soul and know your feelings by how you look at her. Tell her with your eyes what your mouth may not be able to say.

+ Stroke her face and hair. Push her hair off her face. Hold her face as you kiss. Practice the art of light touching—we love it! I know you do too! Use the back of your hand to stroke, as well as fingertips.

+ Many women love being kissed deliciously all over. Try the neck, shoulders, ears, etc. Since we're all different, vary your stimulation above the breasts. Use gentle, lingering kisses. Some of us like it when your tongue darts in and out of our ear and around our neck. Some don't. Gauge her response. Some of us don't like being licked, but you won't know unless you ask or try it.

+ Enjoy her standing up. Start with a loving hug, stroking her back, her hair, and anything else innocuous that moves you.

FOREPLAY APPETIZERS

Foreplay appetizers involve more intimate moves. They increase relaxation and stimulation. Mix and match these juicy tidbits—they'll intensify the heat:

- Undress her slowly. Milk it. Kiss and caress as you remove her clothes. Encourage her to do the same to you. The slower you go, the more anticipation you'll both feel.

- Do sensual stripteases for each other.

- Give her a foot massage. The feet are very sensual. Rub, suck, tickle, fondle, make love to her feet, unless it makes her uncomfortable. It usually relaxes us.

- A sensual massage is delicious for both sexes. Take turns. Use oil and work her body from head to toe, literally. Give her tingles by gently rubbing/tickling her back and arms, letting your lips and tongue follow your fingers, before applying oil. Don't forget hands and feet. Save hot spots for last.

- Try body paint in different flavors. It can be licked off when you're done drawing a masterpiece on each other's bodies. Trace the lines with your tongue.

- Take a sensual shower. Light candles. Wash each other with your fingers. Run your hands up and down each other's slippery bodies, making eye contact.

- Dry hump her. Kiss her tenderly while slowly gyrating the lower half of your body against her. Let her feel how turned on you are without making other sexual moves. Enjoy the anticipation and let her wonder when you'll go for more.

Foreplay as the Main Course

Spend an evening just doing foreplay. Take a sensual shower. Light candles, put on soft music, and sip wine or herbal tea. Lightly touch every inch of each other's bodies standing up. Gently run your hands up and down as you face each other naked. Kiss lips, shoulders, faces, necks, and ears. Look into her eyes while doing this. Eventually lie down facing each other. Do everything very slowly—

savoring every touch and tingle; feeling your partner's soul as you look into her eyes; letting your body respond to this sensuality without rushing. Use a technique I call feathering. Imagine your hand as a feather. Touch her breasts lightly as your hands feather her body. Ask her to do it to you. Feather each other's genitals. From here you can venture in different directions—masturbate yourselves with one hand, continuing to feather each other; masturbate each other; use your hands or mouths to finish it off.

This can be an incredibly sensual experience, making you feel closer to your partner than intercourse does. I recommend it with someone you have loving feelings for. Your partner will love the intimacy it creates as it strengthens your connection. It can create an explosive orgasm from the tension. It's fun to try new things. Have intercourse later.

♨ Hot Tip

Practice a very tender touch on yourself. Lightly brush your arm, until it feels sensual. Practice until you perfect it. Use it all over your partner's body. It will drive most women into submission.

GETTING TO THE "MAIN COURSE"

Chapter 13 goes into detail about our hot spots and how to work them. Use them to find ways to heat us up to the next level. The goal of foreplay should be to have fun and enjoy the wonders of each other's body. Start with the snacks, hors d'oeuvres, and appetizers. Amy wrote that when a man makes love to her, she likes him to "kiss me, then touch me all over my body. I prefer him to wait to touch my clitoris or vagina until he has me good and worked up. At that point, I'm ready for sex in minutes." If we're warmed up, we'll respond more when you touch our hotter spots.

The first time you make love to a woman, start slowly. We can always tell you by our actions if we want you to speed up. We love tenderness. Many of you expressed confusion about what kind of foreplay we need and how much is enough. Ask! If you let her know you want to please her, she'll get comfortable giving instructions. Incorporate suggestions from the next chapters and see how she responds. Remember—SEX IS SUPPOSED TO BE FUN!

13 ROAD MAP TO HOT SPOTS: WORKING THE BUTTONS THAT TURN HER ON

You're about to make love to her for the first time, and you want to satisfy her. There's been lots of touching. You're undressed and ready to go further. You play with her breasts—caress, kiss, do the romantic things I recommended. She seems ready. The time has come—finding her clit. You tentatively put your hand between her legs and hope she responds as you grope around, rubbing the general vicinity of the clit, looking for the right spot. You hate the doubt you feel as you wonder if you actually found it or she's faking. ❧

You can be the best lover possible! By following my map you can learn to find every hot spot on a woman's body and work it well. There are many aspects to being a great lover besides having super "mechanics." Enthusiasm is contagious! We respond well to a man who lovingly does what he can to please and enjoys it. Encourage your partner to say what she wants. Focus on giving her pleasure, not orgasms. If she comes, that's terrific. I can be satisfied without an orgasm but do enjoy them. When a lover says he wants to max out my pleasure, I'll gladly surrender and see what happens. Many women are happy with an all-out effort to make us come, as long as an orgasm isn't mandatory. Once you're in a comfortable relationship, she may relax more and go for it.

Since many women are inhibited, some techniques may be scary or offensive. If we don't understand how something is acceptable, we're afraid to try. Go slowly if your woman is uptight about anything but the missionary position. Wait for a good comfort level. Ask out of bed how she feels about various activities. Let her know what you'd like to try but respect her boundaries. If she refuses everything, ask her to go to counseling with you or accept that you may not be compatible.

Working our hot spots is more active foreplay. True foreplay should be all the romantic gestures that get us into a relaxed and sexy mood. Playing with the hot spots in this chapter is "main play." Cal agrees, "Foreplay gets me as hot as it does women. I search for new spots and ways to please them." *Never forget* that foreplay can be absolutely delicious as the main course. The appetizers were in Chapter 12. This chapter is the meal. The dessert—intercourse—is in Chapter 14. When we're done feasting on everything else, we can have dessert. Sometimes we don't need dessert because the meal was so satisfying. I encourage you to explore each other's bodies and look for even more hot spots as you feast!

There are many ways to touch, lick, suck, and work your partner's body to drive her to the greatest heights of pleasure. This chapter is a road map to our hot spots and what you can do to them. Mix and match like a Chinese food menu. Try each at least once to find a combo that works. Then create what I call your own CLB for your present lady. A CLB is a Custom Lovemaking Blueprint geared specifically to what works for your lover. Plot out all of the erogenous zones, pressure points, and techniques that give her pleasure. Use this blueprint to build the foundation of the hottest sex possible between you. You can't use it on anyone else since it's custom designed for her. Find out what she likes and add it to her CLB as you go. It should include everything that turns her on and all her hot spots.

Anatomy of a Good Lover

Does one take lessons or develop skills? Most of us agree—a great lover is one who doesn't think he knows everything, one who goes with the flow and shows enthusiasm. Skills without passion don't cut it. Yes, some women just want an orgasm and don't care about the rest. But a lot more of us need a lover who cares about our feelings, who explores us as an individual, and who lets us know that our pleasure is his pleasure. You can be the best lover your partner ever had. It starts with wanting to please her. Learn the basics of how her body works, locate her hot spots, create a CLB for her, and you're set!

🔥 **Hot Tip**

Have her lay back in bed and graze her body with your fingertips from head to toe. Then use your lips, just brushing them against her skin.

GOOD LOVER 101

If you want to be a great lover, start by accepting that each of us is an individual with different needs. Your body and roads to orgasm are less complex than ours. You will settle for less and come from less. When we settle for less we don't come. Lynn said, "Many of us don't make it easy for you to be good lovers—we can't tell you specifics." We're great communicators, except in bed. We may know what feels good but can't identify what's being done since we can't see. Try all my suggestions to find those she loves. There's no right or wrong way to touch a woman. If she gives you clues, great. Otherwise, experiment on your own until you get a good reaction. Stay with it.

Get rid of preconceived notions! Don't judge us all by women before us. Guys I interviewed said they knew from experience that women didn't like this or that—I wanted to say, "Wrong! I'd love that done to me!"

A good lover isn't afraid to ask for directions. It's frustrating to communicate if you don't listen. We need different approaches to see what we like and you may continue using the same one whether it works or not. The best lover is one who asks what we like and makes us comfortable sharing or admitting we're not sure, AND who doesn't just stick to the one way he's used to.

Those of you with established techniques won't please us as much as those of you who experiment to see what we like. You "skilled lovers" have a practiced routine. How can you make love to me without treating me as an individual? Encourage your partner to guide you. Create a custom delivery with a CLB. Asking for directions, and *listening,* can make you a first-class lover! Seek and ye shall find! Paula said in frustration:

I think women have a difficult time telling their lover what they want in bed, afraid we'll hurt their feelings if we criticize. But how else will they figure it out? They are not mind readers. Men are pretty black and white with their buddies. I've expressed my desire for more kissing to my current lover but he still doesn't kiss me. I can't get through to him. Our lovemaking has become so routine without foreplay per se. I need to say it again.

I don't understand why so many men stop kissing when they get us into bed, but it happens frequently. Women complain about it often. If you care about her, it seems logical that you'd want to kiss a lot. The more you kiss her, the more relaxed and responsive she can become. Enjoy it!

GOOD LOVER 201

You can learn to be a good lover. If you sincerely care for someone, an expression of feelings *and* a desire to please her preempts skills. A comfortable, loving relationship means more to many of us. Hot sex can develop from a warm and loving connection. It doesn't often work in reverse. Help us along. Sex can heat up quickly as you learn the routes and trust grows. Then she'll be more receptive.

Great, exquisite, mind-blowing sex is less about technique and more about attitude. When I asked women to describe great sex, they were more enthusiastic about the comfort of the sexual interaction and intimacy with their lover. When we feel relaxed, safe, and loved, almost anything you do has the power to make us feel good. Educate yourselves about our bodies and sensitive hot spots to enhance sex. But without an emotional connection, many of us won't respond to even the greatest skills. When we feel emotionally connected, our arousal is heightened.

Sharing intimacy enhances pleasure. It shouldn't be just for the bedroom. Use my suggestions to get connected, and feel intimacy wherever you are together. It fuels our fires. The closer we feel to you, the more we'll open up when intimacy leads to the bedroom. Working on the connection out of bed makes us most receptive to your touch. Remember, so much of sex is in our heads.

Open yourself to the passion I spoke of earlier. Allow your

feelings and excitement to show. We love men who don't hold back. When we hear you express pleasure, it motivates us to put even more effort into pleasing you. Give us a groan or two, boys! The more pleasure you express, the more you'll get. If she knows what she's doing is working, she'll work it more. We love to please. Pleasure noises relax and reassure us—confirmations that you like what we're doing. Say how good she makes you feel. You'll get a hotter chick in return! We want to know you're hot for us. As trust grows, try being more uninhibited. Encourage us to do the same. Let go for yourself. It's a wonderful feeling!

GOOD LOVER 301

Okay, sweethearts. Do you want to please your partner? Do you want her to stop faking orgasms because she's having real ones? The key to great sex is understanding the power of our love button—the clitoris. Women complain that MANY of you neglect this tiny spot with the capacity to give so much pleasure. They implored me to emphasize the importance of identifying and working our clits well. Many women say they only like sex for the cuddling. They might change their minds with a guy who stimulated their clit effectively.

Clitoral stimulation is responsible for a large majority of our orgasms. It's the key to our sexual pleasure. Yet one woman after another complained that many of you spend time on everything but. Become a clit expert! Understand, respect, and revere how important a clit is and what it can do! Clits serve only one function—giving us orgasms. Help it do its job!

Clits are hard to find but worth a search. Once you locate your partner's, go back to it over and over. It's always in the same place so it just takes one major excavation to uncover it. After exploring and discovering what stimulation gives her pleasure, add it to her CLB. Guys, pleasing us isn't brain surgery! Anyone can do it. You own the tools—your lips, tongue, fingers, penis. Go on a mission to pinpoint her clit and try every technique in this book until you discover what she enjoys (more on this will follow). Etch this in your brain—*the clit is it!*

Hot Spots Are Everywhere!

Every nook and cranny of our bodies can be a hot spot. Each of us responds to different ones, so stimulate them all until you find those to include in her CLB. Watch her response to each. The possibilities are endless. Don't make the decision by one time. She may not respond at first. As she relaxes more with you after you've had sex for a while, her body may open up and respond more. Encourage her to let you know when you do something she likes.

Personalize Sex	
DON'T SAY	DO SAY
"I love sex."	"I love being inside of you."
"This feels great."	"Making love to you feels great."
"I'm getting so hot."	"You're making me so hot."

THE WONDERS OF OUR BREASTS

Many of us love having our breasts played with. But women complain that many of you just grab on and squeeze before moving to juicier spots. Want to get many of us juiced? Make love to our breasts. Both the areola (the darker ring around the nipple) and nipple get easily aroused. The stimulation can be potent to some of us. Jennifer said, "If a man squeezes my nipples in his fingers, and then sucks them hard, occasionally biting, I can come." Some of us like to be licked and sucked gently and can't handle hard sucking or biting. Some of us like rougher handling or both. The size of her breasts isn't related to her response to stimulation.

When you first make love to her, start gently unless she wants more. Play with her breasts, squeezing, kissing, and licking them. Create a CLB for her breasts. Use your fingers to play with her nipples. Rub the nipple with two or more fingers. Pinch it softly and then a little harder as you gauge her response. Ask if she'd like more pressure. Moisten your fingers with saliva or cream for a better sensation.

How do we like our breasts sucked? Many ways of course! Kiss them. Lightly make circles around her nipples with your tongue. Put your mouth over a nipple and suck gently. Flick your tongue on it at the same time. Ask for feedback. Suck just the nipple or as much as you get in your mouth. Some of us like them sucked hard, some gentle. Some like to be sucked like a nursing baby. Bite it softly. ASK, "Would you like me to bite harder or is this better?" Some of us like it so hard you're scared you'll hurt it. If we say so, do it.

Go from one breast to the other. Hold them together for alternating with your tongue. Suck one breast—use your hand on the other. Some of us like your penis rubbed on our breasts. Enjoy playing and add what makes us squeal to our CLB. By the way, your own breasts are hot spots too. Stimulate your nipples when you masturbate to see if it affects you. Let her lick and suck them.

The Body as an Erogenous Zone

Every inch of a woman's body can be an erogenous zone if you touch sensually. Obvious spots will make us respond quicker, but try them all. Theresa said, "Men forget there are parts of the female anatomy other than the breast and vagina." Nerve endings all over our body respond to your hands, mouth, and tongue. When I read that armpits were erogenous zones, I told my boyfriend to skip deodorant after a shower and he loved the stimulation.

More subtle spots work better for those in tune with their erotic side. Initiate her slowly. Stimulate her earlobes, neck, inner thighs, palms, belly button, and lower back. Cal recommends, "Gently kiss her fingertips, palm of her hand, base of her neck, crook of her elbow or knee." Fingers and toes are incredibly sensual. Lick and suck them when she's showered. Sucking toes sensually can be intense. Not everything will do it for every woman. There are enough places to explore to add dimension to our CLB. Mary advised, "Touch her whole body. Everything can be erogenous. Be a conquistador, so to speak. She's naked, appreciate that." Start exploring with a feathery touch like I spoke of in the last chapter. That can make her more conducive for more active touching. Tender, feathery grazing of her body should make her purr. Then you can explore deeper.

Pinpointing the Clit and Working It

You're about to have sex—she opens her legs for stimulation. You know her clit is somewhere so you rub the vicinity between her legs. Why not? Other women accepted that. You figure if you rub her enough, she'll get wet and you can jump on. You move your hand randomly around her vagina. She seems more moist so you assume you hit the spot and keep working that area. She tries moving your hand but why mess with a sure thing? So you keep your rhythm. But when you move to enter her, she tells you not to bother until you work her clit over. You're confused. Weren't you doing that? ~

Many of you are clueless about the clitoris. Unless you've been with a woman who guided, you may still practice what I call mushing—putting your hand over the vagina, rubbing, and praying for the best. I've asked past lovers if they knew where my clit was and got sheepish "I hope so's" and "probably not's." One macho type boasted, "I know exactly where." It was hard not saying, "Then why don't you touch it?" Remember—*the clit is it!*

GENITAL ITINERARY

Have you explored between our legs without sex? Do it with your partner. Check us out with a mirror. The clit is at the front of the vaginal opening, just above where our lips (labia) meet. Only the tip is visible. It's been described as looking like a pea. It's the only pea-like thing there so you should recognize it. Some doctors say a clit is like a mini penis—with the same sensitivity as yours. When aroused, it swells into an erection too. Jesse said, "Women's parts are in different shapes and sizes. It's an adventure."

The clit is covered by a hood. Sometimes it pokes its horny head out on its own. Sometimes you have to pull the hood back to find it. Pull the skin around her clit gently up toward her tummy with two fingers. It usually lifts the hood up to reveal the tip. Sometimes it's hidden more and you have to find a way to pull the skin back to get to it. It's worth a search when you see the results!

To confuse you more, our clits can be fickle. Many of us have a more sensitive side or one spot works best. Try left and right, asking your partner which gives more sensation. Hot spots on the clit aren't always consistent. What gets us going may stop feeling good and you may have to move around to find another spot. This is normal. After an orgasm some of us are so sensitive that we can't be touched immediately. You may have to give her a breather before continuing. All women are multiorgasmic but not all of us can handle multiple orgasms. If she says "no more," stay off the clit.

Touching Our Love Button

You can do many things to our clit with your fingers. Experiment the first time and ask for input. Don't be discouraged if you get none. When rubbing a clit, try different ways to see how she responds. Rub it up and down, from side to side, and in a circular motion. Different women mentioned all of these as things they liked. Experiment. Ask her to put her hand on yours and guide your moves as you stimulate her. Let her use your hand as an instrument until you get the right motion, pressure, and speed.

When you work the clit, ask your partner to use her own fingers to pull the lips aside and expose it for you. If she masturbates she probably knows the most effective way to get its little head to come to the surface. It leaves you with your hands free to explore other parts of her and gives her more control over where you go and how much needs to be uncovered.

Use your fingers on and around the vaginal area and clit. Some women like pressure right on it. Some are too sensitive and can't be touched directly, so rub around it. The clit should be moist. Stick your finger inside your partner's vagina to get natural lubrication, or use saliva or a lubricant. There are many ways to touch with your fingers. Lea said, "Make circles around the clitoris to tease. Then wet your finger and rub it up and down. Alternate between that and your palm but always nail the clitoris. When orgasm is close go back to fingers up and down." Claire advises, "Find and fondle the clit. Rub it gently between two fingers and then use your thumb, alternating between putting pressure on it and rubbing back and forth. Insert a finger or two, always keeping a thumb or palm on the clit with steady rhythm." We like fingers inside! Al suggested:

Put your index and pointer fingers inside her vagina palm up. Bend them so they hit the G-spot. Practice going in and out of her vigorously in a way that the top of your palm slaps her clit on each move. It takes coordination but once you get the knack, you'll drive her crazy. I often let my girl lay back. I get on my knees in front of her and slam her with the various parts of my hand. The bent fingers simulate the G-spot. It gets women worked up for other things.

Fingers, fingers, fingers. Many of us can't have too many stimulating us. Insert one or two inside. Work them around slowly. Go shallow. Go deep. Explore us slowly. Use two fingers and do an imitation of your penis during intercourse. Go in and out quickly, hitting the clit with your hand. Some of us like it rough. Try different angles. Have fun with it.

Tasting Our Love Button

Women report the most effective way to give us an orgasm is with oral sex. Many of you swear it works every time. Cal agrees, "Oral sex is sometimes, if not always, as wonderful as intercourse. I believe it can be more satisfying, especially for women." There's lots of variety with oral sex. For many, many, many of us, there's nothing like a tongue. It can do what nothing else can. It's more flexible than a penis or finger and has natural lubricant—saliva. It can reach little crevices and bitty hot spots much easier. So many of us swear by oral sex that it's a pity for you not to indulge us. Yet many of you don't.

Some of you complain you don't like giving oral sex because of our scent. Bob said, "I love the aroma of my wife's pussy and spend lots of time between her legs. I love lapping as I breathe her in. She's clean and I lick it up!" Jesse advises, "To make sure she's clean, give her a bath. Women love that. Get her soapy and clean her. That can turn her on." He added that men's testosterone and women's estrogen kicks off pheromones, which create a natural scent for sexual attraction. When you lose yourself in sensuality, the scent of sex is an aphrodisiac. Jesse said, "If you don't like it, you don't know what you're missing."

GREAT ORAL SEX

Start oral sex by kissing your way down to her genitals. Tenderly make love to us between our legs. First kiss our most private parts the way you'd kiss our face. Flick the tip of your tongue on the edge of her clit or a spot she responds to. Some of us like it right on the clit; some prefer licking around it. Tease lightly with only your tongue. David said, "I start making big circles with my tongue. They get smaller until I'm on the clit. Then I go round and round on it." Watch her reaction. Some women like being flicked from side to side; some said up and down. Some just want to be flicked every way! Use your fingers at the same time you're using your tongue. Either use a thumb on her clit along with your tongue, or go in and out of her vagina with your fingers. Press on our G-spot (see next the section). Many of us love two fingers deeply embedded in our vagina as you lick, or use them going in and out fast, complementing your tongue.

 Sexy Tip

Rub the palm of your hand over her clit as you kiss. During oral sex, stop, palm her clit, and press. Gauge the pressure by her reaction.

Create a precision clit stimulator with your tongue. David said, "Keep the tongue rigid and flick it fast on the clit." It helps hit the mark accurately. Other guys suggested making your tongue a hard pointy tip and working her clit like that. Or let her sit on your face, with one knee on either side of your head or resting on your shoulders. This gives her control over how you stimulate her. She can guide your mouth to spots that create the best sensations.

Some of you dig your face into our vaginal area, licking and sucking everywhere. Some of you use your tongue like a mini penis going in and out of the vagina. Alex said, "I don't put my tongue all the way inside. It's more the opening to the inside that's sensitive." There are few nerve endings inside but many of us love having your mouth there, as long as you pay attention to the clit! When you suck the clit, use your tongue too. Jesse described a technique many women said they love but weren't sure what was done:

Put your mouth around the area of the clit like a little suction cup. The concept is to be like a plunger. Get the clit in your mouth, hold the skin back if needed, and suck it like a kid sucking on a baby bottle nipple. Once you have the clit in your mouth, hold it there sucking it in and use your tongue to flick on her clit, back and forth like a pendulum.

As our excitement builds, we need consistent rhythm, motion, and pressure. Constant change-ups drive many of us crazy. We may be close and just need a bit more, but you slow down, change direction, or do something to break the train of our fragile orgasm. Be fluid in your moves. Some of us need just the right rhythm or we lose it. You may speed up or slow down a bit too much for us to maintain the arousal we need to reach an orgasm. At first we may like more variety. Slower, faster, softer, more pressure, different directions can add to our turn-on. But when we're getting closer, consistent stimulation puts us over the top faster.

Try sex toys. Ask your partner how she feels about a vibrator. Small battery-operated ones are easy to maneuver around your body. Experiment with different kinds to see what works for her. Use your tongue on one side of her clit and a small vibrator on the other. Use the vibrator when your tongue gets tired. Alternate stimulations and include fingers too. Let her use it on you. A vibrator is a massager—it stimulates. Try using it all over each other's bodies first.

The G-Spot

Does the G-spot exist? It depends on who you ask! Some experts say "yes." Some refute it. Some women say they have one. Some are more clueless than you. Those who've experienced its pleasure assure me it's worth finding.

The G-spot is located on the outer wall of the vagina, about one and a half or two inches up. Jesse described it as a little shelf against the outside wall and you can feel the ridge inside if you look for it. Leo said it feels like a soft round spot. He said he feels it swell up as he massages it. Put your finger(s) inside, slightly bent, with your palm face up. Stimulation varies. Let her tell you. Explore the area with a finger. Gray advised:

Put a finger or two inside her with your hand facing up toward her belly. Rub the area about one to two inches in. It's hard to describe the spot. Each woman is unique. Explore. Listen to how she reacts to it. I apply firm pressure when I hit the spot. I massage it too. One woman said it made her feel like she had to pee, but it passed. Some like it more than others. Those who love it say it gives them orgasms that are more deep and intense.

Ian recommends, "Manually stimulate. Some like fast—some slow—some just a steady press, firmly. Some like very slight pressing and then rotate 180 degrees and go for oral stimulation at the same time, some anal and oral and hit the G-spot—if the police arrive, you've gone too far!" To intensify a G-spot orgasm, either you or your partner can press on her lower tummy just along the line of her pubic bone as your finger massages her G-spot. It puts pressure on it from outside and can speed an orgasm. Glenda recommends, "Work back and forth, stimulating the G-spot until an orgasm is almost there and then switch to the clit. Do it a few times. Bring us to the edge and switch." Watch her explode when you let her come! As you work the G-spot, stimulate her clit with your other hand or your tongue simultaneously. Press your finger against it as you stimulate other parts. Custom G-spot stimulation is a great tool to add to her CLB!

Let's not forget you, you sweet guys who want to please us. Do you know that you have a G-spot too? It's centered in your prostate, which makes it a bit less likely that she'll search for it since that's in your tush. A finger stimulating the inside of the anus when an orgasm is approaching can intensify it for both men and women. Many women say they love that kind of anal stimulation and would do it to you. Some would make a face and refuse to discuss it.

Try a little anal stimulation on her first, with her permission. Ask her to do it to you if she's comfortable. You don't have to go that far up. Press down just inside the opening toward her clit. She may guide you. An easier way for her to intensify your orgasm is to rub your perineum. That's the area of skin between your genitals and tush, that usually has no hair. If she massages or presses on it when you're nearing orgasm, it could intensify it dramatically. She'll have to experiment to see what stimulation feels best.

FEMALE EJACULATION

You're not the only ones who ejaculate. Some of us do too! During an orgasm, liquid may come out a little or in a gusher like your ejaculation. Female ejaculation hasn't been studied for long so there isn't too much concrete info about it except that it's natural. Some of you say your biggest turn-on is getting a geyser out of her. It often happens during or after an orgasm when you rub her G-spot. We may get scared and think we're peeing on you but that's not usually the case. Some studies show that the clear fluid isn't urine, though some might be mixed in. Either way it's washable.

BEST ROUTES TO ORGASM

Since many of us only come from oral stimulation, here's advice from women who love it. Pay attention to our noise, body language, and how wet we get to know when you're on the money.

Merelee: I love being sucked hard and then having the tip of his tongue go fast over just my clit. Keep the mouth off at this point. I just want to feel tongue.

Jeri: Get a good rhythm with your tongue and finger and keep it. I need a constant steady stimulation—not slower then faster then slower. If something is working, stick with it.

Carla: Start off gently and build up as my excitement does. As you hear me feeling turned on, increase the speed and the pressure on my clit.

Gia: We like being touched lightly and slowly. Work your way to faster. We like being teased, like you do. Vary stimulation between your tongue, fingers, lips, and palm.

Judy: I like if a man goes down on me and puts his fingers in me at the same time. If he had two more hands, I'd like him to fondle my nipples too but that's four arms. Oh well!

Betty: I like a tongue to touch my clitoris and stop and then start until I'm there.

Georgia: Don't go down on me like a starving man. Some guys dig in so deep it's like searching for gold. Keep it light, especially at first. Start off gently licking, kissing, and teasing. As I get hotter, focus on my clitoris. That's how to strike gold!

Linda: I need you to start slowly and increase the pressure as I get aroused. I'm a musician and to me an orgasm is like building to a crescendo. Many men think they have to go at high speed all the time. Not true. Steady is better. A nice steady rhythm and slowly lick—as we get more excited, touch harder and faster. Make us sound like a symphony!

Shana: I love being able to lay back and have my guy do me. From head to toe and then head for the clit. I love being treated like a goddess that way. When he finishes eating me out and I've had several orgasms, I put lots into reciprocating.

I asked for your special techniques of getting your partner to orgasm:

James: My girl goes easier when I let her know how much looking at her body turns me on. Lots of compliments put most women at ease.

Clayton: It's that clit. You've gotta learn to work it. When you find out how she likes it and give her plenty of stimulation, wait for her body to pulsate.

Buck: I kiss her a lot—I mean a lot. The more I kiss her, the more she relaxes. The more she relaxes, the more chance of orgasms. I kiss her till she melts and succumbs to me.

Ian: Some like oral, some manual, some slow, some fast, some very light, some heavy touch, some like to have it sucked, some licked. Play fair and try it all. See what drives them through the headboard.

Jack: I make love to every inch of her body, with attention to sensitive spots like nipples, fingers, inner thighs and then between her legs. I kiss everything with the same passion and attention I give her lips. She goes quick by the time I use my tongue on her clitoris.

Seth: Massages work great, especially with sensual oil. I slowly massage her whole body. When I'm finished, she's in another world and so loose she can have several orgasms.

Jeff: I tease a lot with my tongue. I put it inside her and play with her clit. Then I use a finger. I tease with the tip at different speeds, then slowly work it in and out. I'll use another finger in her butt.

John described:

I like to kiss all around before kissing, licking, and sucking her. Then I push my tongue in deeper and run it up and down the length of her pussy, alternating between the outside on one side, the outside on the other, then in the middle. I spread her lips wide with my fingers and start tonguing her clit. After a bit I suck her clit and a good-sized amount of her lips firmly into my mouth. While still sucking firmly I run my tongue around and over her clit a bit faster as she gets anxious to come. As I'm sucking her and tonguing her clit I move one hand up and squeeze her tits, pulling her nipples. I take the other hand and stick two or three fingers into her vagina and move them around keeping pressure on different sides of the rim.

Jesse described what his father, Bay, called "Triple Whammy":

It takes coordination. Get her on her back. Don't dive in right away. Kiss her around the ears, back of neck. Work your way down her neck and around her shoulders. Lick around the nipples. Gently bite down on each and roll your tongue around. Ask exactly what she likes. Kiss your way around her belly button. Start on the hair around her pubic area. That's real sensitive. Go inside her thighs. Keep your hands moving. Get spit between your thumb and pointer finger. Reach up—squeeze and roll her nipples around. Find her clit. She can help you out by pulling the skin back with two fingers to expose it. Lick the clit and pussy gently. Straddle her right leg. Keep rubbing her nipple with your moist left hand and put the middle finger of your right hand in her pussy near the bottom. Get a finger going. Gently put your finger in and out, just a half-inch in, real quick, like you were tapping something with the tip of your finger. Once she starts getting moist and wet, lick the hell out of her clit real fast, like a snake's tongue, gently flutter it and flick it all around. You can suck it a bit. Keep playing with her nipple, using your finger with short little strokes, as fast as you can and as she holds the clit open, lap the heck out of it, all at the same time! If she wants an orgasm, she'll have it from this triple whammy!

Communicate. Emphasize "I'm asking because I want to give you pleasure." Eventually you should know enough to create her CLB. Encourage her to be freer. Suggest she stroke her body. She can stimulate her breasts or lightly touch herself all over while you do her genitals. Leann said, "I used to lay back and settle for what a man did. Now I've learned to touch my own body—my genitals, stomach, nipples—while he's doing his thing to me. That ensures all bases are covered!"

You want great sex? Satisfy us first and we'll bend over backward or forward or sideways to please you. Harry said, "When you please a woman first, you won't have to worry about hot sex. She's receptive to everything." Ian advises:

Touch easy until you get to know what makes them push into or crave more touch; they will move their body to the degree of stimulation they want. If you learn to read their language—without regard for your pleasure first—she will be insatiable because she feels that her pleasure is the single most important thing to you in the world. Look out for what she gives back—times ten—she will be on a mission to please if you make sure you were her very best!

If you're in a long-term relationship, get to know your partner's body well. As you treasure each part, she'll open up more. As you take the time to make love to her as a precious commodity, she'll hopefully want to do the same for you. When you're each in complete tune with each other's pleasure and passion, you sweethearts will discover where the term "making love" came from.

14

HOT SEX:
HOW TO BE HER DREAM LOVER

S he seems to melt as her face is kissed. Every technique seems to heat her up more. Under the sheets she moans, purrs, and arches her back in what must be a giant orgasm. Afterward, she expresses her great satisfaction and an undying need to continue making love. It would be so wonderful if you were the man and she were your partner. But that's not the case. You're in the movies and the lovers are on screen. You wonder if giving your partner that much pleasure is possible in real life. If only you could find a way to be the kind of lover women lust after. ~

You see it in movies. People speak of it. You want it too. HOT SEX. Is mutually satisfying lovemaking that takes each partner to pleasure extremes possible in the real world? YES! YES! YES! Let's tie what you've already learned and the lessons in this chapter together to create the best CLB.

Creating a blueprint for the hottest sex possible entails trying all the tools and putting them into the right formula for both of you. Many of you don't feel confident as a lover. Do you think knowing how to make love is something you're born with? No! You all start somewhere. Some of you had a more experienced woman teach you. More of you said your main education was from porno flicks.

Sex education videos don't teach everything but do provide instruction. Trial and error with a new partner is the best teacher. If you're in a long-term relationship, communicate and experiment openly. Read books and watch videos with your partner. There are an unlimited number of ways to make love. Mix and match to keep the excitement of making love to the same partner high. And never forget—*the clit is it!*

Making Her More Comfortable Giving Oral Sex

You've given her lots of foreplay. Your manhood is standing at attention in her face. She's moaning as you continue pleasuring her. You're aroused and raring for action, yet she doesn't move to reciprocate. You shift positions so she can feel your penis's throbbing head, and still she ignores it. You want her to take you in her mouth but don't have the nerve to ask. So you gently try pulling her south of the border. She resists and you pull harder. Eventually she gets the message and halfheartedly sucks your penis. If you come in her mouth, she may never do it again. Why are so many women difficult about oral sex? ～

You consistently express dissatisfaction with the quality, frequency, and enthusiasm behind the oral sex you've received. You have a hard time convincing or encouraging women to give you satisfying head. Studies show that when men pay for sex, blowjobs are the most requested sexual act. Many of you are thrilled to put your mouths on our genitals and pleasure us to tears. Why are so many of us reluctant to reciprocate with the same pleasure?

MORE CONDUCIVE TO SUCK

Many of you think only a very small percentage of women really enjoy giving oral sex. You're not far off. Many of us like it because we enjoy pleasing you, not because we enjoy sucking you. Remember, our sexuality has been stifled. Many of us grew up believing that putting a penis in one's mouth is dirty. Put yourself in our places. If you've never been with a man, you can't image what it's like to have a penis in your mouth. If you're large, it's hard to maneuver it comfortably. Many of us have gagged when a guy thrust hard.

You want us to worship your penis, to lovingly lick and suck it. More often, we complain about getting tired. Many of us don't like swallowing, much to the chagrin of most of you. We want to be warned before you come. Knowing we want to pull back when you want us to stay put and eagerly swallow your juices takes the edge off your pleasure. The taste of semen varies. What you eat affects it. Since some of you don't get oral sex often, when you do, you hold your erection as long as possible, which makes us even less inclined next time.

There's no easy solution to our aversion to sucking you. Talk to her openly. Tell her what oral sex means to you. This program may be hard to change. I asked women what you can do to make them more comfortable. To start with, BE CLEAN! Don't you expect us to be? If she complains that your pubic hair irritates her face, use conditioner on it when you shower. Be sure to let her know you're enjoying it. Your sounds of pleasure will encourage her, Silence makes her look up a lot for signs that she's doing it in a way that pleases you. That keeps her from relaxing. Make noise. Tell her how good she makes you feel. That will spur her on! Jenna said, "Make a lot of noise. Do NOT shove my head down."

Women also emphasized the importance of allowing us our own pace. Some of you push your partner's head onto your penis when she doesn't want to. That's a turnoff. Mary said, "Don't EVER, EVER, push down a woman's head when she's giving you head. That is utterly degrading." Don't force it if she's not ready. Let her find her own way. I thought you'd appreciate Theresa's answer. "I enjoy giving oral sex to a man very much. To me, it's the most generous thing I can do and it is probably as much a turn-on for me as it is for him. I masturbate and usually bring myself to orgasm while giving it. Just be clean!"

Sexy Tip

While she's going down on you, say her name several times. "Oh Jennifer, that feels sensational." "You are so good to me, Jennifer." Pleasure statements with her name will motivate her to keep going."

SUCKING IN SMALL DOSES

Most of you indicated you'd love *any* contact between your genitals and her mouth. Let her get used to oral sex by encouraging her to lick and kiss you lovingly. Suggest that she think of oral sex as making love to your genitals. Let her fondle and taste. Don't rush her. Let her get used to having oral contact without taking your penis in her mouth. Ask her to use her tongue lightly along the ridge of the head of your penis on the underside. You know where I mean. A light tongue feels good and gives her a chance to have oral contact without going too fast. If you let her get used to putting her mouth on your genitals without actually sucking it, she may give you what you want when she is comfortable and experiences how much you enjoy it. Let her know how much through words or by moaning. She'll want to do more.

Many of us will eventually take you in our mouth if we can do it at our own pace. Show her how to use her hand with her mouth. Show her how to keep her hand near the base of your penis and move it up and down in sync with her mouth. Keep water nearby so she has enough saliva. Don't push her to take too much of your penis in your mouth at once. You don't want her to gag.

Many of you like simultaneous oral sex. It's harder for us to concentrate on receiving pleasure and giving you good head at the same time. You don't want us to bite you if we get carried away with pleasure. We may not allow ourselves to get as turned on as when we're being served solo. Most women prefer to give and get oral sex separately. Ask.

If she agrees, there are many ways to mutually pleasure each other's genitals by mouth. You can lie on your back with your partner over you. We feel more comfortable like this because we can control how deep you go in our mouth. Pull her vagina down over your mouth or lift your head. Put pillows under your head. Depending on the angle, you may be able to play with her breasts in this position. Or try her on the bottom. This position makes some of us nervous that you may thrust too deep. Or, you can lie side by side, using pillows to prop various parts for comfort.

"What Can I Do to Satisfy Her During Intercourse?"

You've just had a very satisfying lovemaking session with your girlfriend. Intercourse was wonderful. You held your erection for quite a while and are pleased with your performance. She seemed to be enjoying it. As you roll over, exhausted from your athletic accomplishments, she asks you if you'd please use your finger or tongue to stimulate her to orgasm. Why didn't it happen when you were inside of her? ~

Studies show that up to 70 percent of us don't have orgasms during intercourse. A majority of women in my classes still find intercourse very satisfying, but need other stimulation to come. The area inside of the vagina isn't too sensitive. The clit still works best for orgasm. Your partner might not come from intercourse alone, but most of us are quite capable of coming that way *with the appropriate stimulation*. Get creative. There's more than one way for a woman to explode while you're inside of her. Since every woman is different, I'll give you plenty of techniques to try that can make intercourse more pleasurable for both of you.

Vaginal versus Clitoral Orgasms

Some women say they experience two different kinds of orgasms, vaginal orgasms (from intercourse) and clitoral ones (from direct stimulation of the clit). The vaginal walls don't have nerve endings that create the sensations for orgasm, except for the area of the G-spot. Those having vaginal ones may get indirect stimulation on their clits. An orgasm with a penis inside feels different because the penis affects our muscle contractions. Vaginal orgasms can come from your penis hitting the G-spot. Does it matter? As long as she's satisfied, why worry where it comes from!

Women often describe vaginal orgasms as "more emotional." Katie said, "A vaginal orgasm feels deeper and fuller, more intense on some levels. They make me feel more emotionally connected to my husband." Stacy is also sure she has two kinds, "I only have vaginal orgasms with men I trust in a serious relationship. Then I feel a vaginal orgasm in my soul." Perhaps the difference is that being inside of us during the orgasms gives us that deeper connection. Again, do labels matter? Whatever works is good.

Developing Your "Clit Radar" System

Develop what I call "clit radar." Always know where her clit is and aim for it in creative ways. Almost all women can go off from enough of the right kind of clit stimulation. Try everything, but if you work the clit too, you'll have the best chance of putting her over the top. Women asked me to repeat this: It astounds them that you do everything BUT stimulate the clit—this is the key to our sexuality!!

How do you activate and maintain your "clit radar"? Make the effort to get a true fix on exactly where your partner's clit is, even if it feels like a major excavation. A clit can be hard to find, but once you do it will always be in the same place. Memorize it. Then—no matter what else you're doing, give it attention. This isn't rocket science. The clit is our tried and true hot spot. It loves stimulation. Working it has the highest odds of giving us an orgasm. That's the button to keep pushing! Affix your radar to it as soon as sex play begins. It can start with a knee between our legs. Before and during intercourse you can rub it with your fingers, palm, tongue, penis, or whatever. Give it lots of stimulation just prior to intercourse. Betty said, "Oral sex right before my husband penetrates me heightens and lengthens my orgasm." It'll get her as primed as possible before you enter. Slippery is nice!

Depending on how far you can reach, use any part of your finger or palm to manipulate our love button. Hopefully by this time you'll have learned how your partner likes to be stroked. During intercourse, you or your partner can use a finger or vibrator on the clit. The key is actually touching her clit, not just the general vicinity. Don't just grope around. Hone your radar and aim for it. Practice locating that little spot. Remember—*the clit is it!* Don't take the attitude that we should be able to come just from feeling you inside. It doesn't always work that way. But, isn't it nice knowing there are things you can do to maximize the possibilities of your partner having an orgasm with you inside of her?

Using angles during intercourse allows you to rub against her clit as you go in and out. I can't be specific since we're all different. Find the way by picturing exactly where the clit is in relation to your position during intercourse. As you thrust your body in, lift it up toward the clit. It's often described as lifting your pelvis up toward hers. Aim your body against the clit as you go in and out. You'll probably need a bit of practice to get the flow but when your partner sees how great it feels, I'm sure she'll be thrilled if you practice on her. Just zoom in on the clit with each move. Your radar will become better and eventually come naturally. I'll give more pointers when I describe individual positions.

SIMULTANEOUS ORGASMS

The simultaneous "ahhh!" What a turn-on to achieve it!

Simultaneous orgasms happen more frequently in the movies than in real life. It's nice when we orgasm at different times. Yours excites us more and ours excites you. Remeber, we can have more than one. With a woman who's willing to allow herself several, you'll have a greater chance of getting one off with her. But, don't get caught in the expectation trap. If you make climaxing at the same time too important, you may get much less pleasure than you could. Relax and enjoy. It may just come naturally. As you and your partner get more attuned to each other's patterns and levels of arousal, you may be able to find your way to one. There are exercises you can do that are found in other books if you want to work on it. I personally don't think sex should be work. It's too much fun!

 Sexy Tip

Undress her slowly, kissing each bit of skin as it gets exposed.

Keeping Your Erection for Longer

Many of you expressed concern about not being able to hold your erection long enough to please us. Some of you have been criticized for coming too soon. I won't lie. Women do complain about men who "don't last long enough." If you come before we've had enough, you can continue stimulating with your mouth or fingers. Sex doesn't have to end because you've had an orgasm. Zach said, "I always say the first orgasm is for me cause that one is quick; the rest are for her." Communication tells you if we'd like you to keep going by other means. There are many reasons you may ejaculate before you'd like to. I'll talk about some of the common ones and give suggestions. It's normal to come quickly during sex. But you may be able to extend your erection, if you choose to.

MINDING YOUR ERECTION

Just as our minds control our orgasms, your minds affect how long you can keep from ejaculating. You may come faster if you've been without sex for a while. Trying to hold it is worse. You've said you may come quickly if we turn you on like crazy. Andy said, "Sometimes I can go at intercourse for ages. But my current girlfriend is so hot that I can barely hold it once I'm inside of her. Knowing it bothers her makes it worse." It can be more mental than physical. Sandy added:

> When I got involved with Keith, he said he loved being inside me so much that he didn't want to come. He'd hold his erection for a long time and said it was longer than ever. When we began having problems out of bed and he was angry, he came in two minutes. It got very frustrating how he could go from one extreme to another. We discussed it and he said he had no idea of why it happened. I think he just didn't care anymore.

What's going on that might keep you from holding your erection longer? Are you tired? Do you bring work-related problems into bed? Is your concern about coming too soon making you come too soon? Is low self-esteem contributing—you're not doing well at work or don't feel good about your body? If any of these fit you, try changing your mindset. You have the power if the cause is mental. Take the pressure off yourself in bed. Learn how to control the timing of your ejaculation instead of worrying about it. Make a conscious effort to last longer. First make sure you don't have a physical problem. I highly recommend you all get checked regularly by a urologist and have your prostate screened. Don't wait until a problem is serious before finding it. You love your penis? Take good care of it!

CONTROLLING EJACULATION

Try delaying ejaculation through masturbation. Instead of whacking off in the bathroom, lie back and pleasure yourself slowly, trying different techniques for touching yourself. Massaging your testicles can feel good. Use both hands some of the time. As you approach an orgasm, slow down and then stop for a ten count or more. Find the right timing. Then start again slowly. This can be carried over to delay an orgasm in bed. Sensual masturbation helps you to get to know your own body. Get used to delaying orgasm by slowing down as it approaches, and then try it with your partner.

Pace yourself during intercourse. Start slowly. If you feel yourself on the brink, slow down a lot or stop a minute. Use this opportunity to kiss her or play with her breasts. We like that kind of diversion. When you're inside, switch from going in and out of her vagina to slowly going from side to side or in circles with your penis. That feels good to both of you. Stir her vagina for a minute as you catch your breath. When you're comfortable with your partner, let her know why you take breaks. Go down on her for a few minutes. Use fingers or a vibrator on her clit to keep her going. When you feel less on the edge of an orgasm, return to intercourse. Stopping and starting can delay an orgasm and can intensify it when it comes! Doing this regularly will improve timing for many of you.

There are whole books with techniques to postpone orgasm if it becomes a serious problem. Here are a few more suggestions that can help. You say changing your position buys time. Stop a minute and focus on your partner. Give her a long, sensual kiss. That can take the focus away from your genitals for a moment and will get her more aroused. When you feel an orgasm approach, slow down with some deep breaths or more slow kisses.

I tell women to do kegel exercises to intensify their orgasm. This means squeezing the muscles you do when you have to pee, there's no bathroom and you have to hold it. Some of you say squeezing these muscles can bring you down a bit. Do these kegels when you're not having sex to strengthen your muscles. That can also give you more control, and better orgasms. Some of you think unsexy thoughts to slow yourself—you picture your boss, the news headlines, the weather forecast. Take pressure off of your testicles by keeping your legs apart. Keeping them together puts pressure on them and can make an orgasm more urgent. Many of you can delay ejaculation if you want to.

The Best Intercourse She's Ever Had

Good sex is loving play. Don't make it too serious. Laugh with your partner if a new position fails. Let her know that you love making love to her and not just to her genitals. Intercourse is a connection for women. Since we tie sex with love, or at least with caring, we can take it more seriously than you. Get a balance between keeping it light and connecting with us on an emotional level.

Some Intercourse Logistics

Respect her boundaries. If you get her to try something new, stop immediately if she asks you to. If you respect what makes her uncomfortable, she may be more likely to try new things again. Intercourse doesn't mean pounding hard with your penis. Many of you think we want it hard and fast. That's fine once she's warmed up, but start slowly and gently, unless she tells you otherwise. Build the intensity as our excitement grows. Mary advised:

> Don't knock her head against the headboard. Stop and move down if you have to. Don't ram your dick in like you're trying to break through a brick wall. Wait until she's wet enough or use some lubrication before trying to jam it in. Kiss her, engage her in foreplay, and at least pretend the actual intercourse isn't the only pleasurable part of the scenario . . . Try to get her off instead of just trying to get off yourself. You have a much better chance of having an orgasm than she does. Keep that in mind and don't be selfish.

Ask what positions she likes and which new ones she'd like to try. Following is a round up of what both sexes said they liked. Try them all at least once if she's game. Be patient about trying new things that might be out of her realm, like anal sex. Some women may be into bondage or other less traditional kinds of sex play and some may refuse to discuss them. If it interests you, ask how she feels. But wait until you know her well before bringing up things that are considered kinky, unless she's let you know she's open-minded.

Give her lots of clitoral stimulation before entering her. Ian said, "It's better to give them an orgasm before intercourse. Then they're more into it." Omar added, "If you want a chance for her to come during intercourse, rub and lick her clit—a lot—first."

Sensations during intercourse vary depending on how much her legs are open or closed. In all positions, the penis goes in deeper when our legs are open. Bending our knees can also allow deeper penetration. This is especially good if your penis is short. What seems to work in stimulating an orgasm for many women is any variation of having our legs together. You hit the clit more. It takes getting used to but her response can be dramatic. Try entering her while she's lying flat on her back with her legs together and straight out. You may have to start out in an easier position for entry and then get your legs on the outside of hers and bring her legs together. This lines your penis up with her clit. Remember—*the clit is it!*

Another variation that women swear by for an orgasm is having her lie flat on top of you with her legs straight behind her. Many women are uncomfortable if they're self-conscious of their weight on you. It's also awkward. Encourage her to work with you on that. Having her legs together during intercourse intensifies muscle tension and increases stimulation to those all-important orgasmic nerve endings. Trying this may not seem natural at first. But your efforts can result in some delicious orgasms. Sharyl attested:

> *I only have an orgasm during intercourse if my legs are closed. I like being on top and keeping my legs closed tight. That's the best if I'm with a guy who works with me on that. The next best is being on the bottom with my legs straight out. It takes a little getting used to and slick moves to do but it's worth the results. I come every time.*

If she's not wet enough, use saliva or a lubricant. Be aware that sometimes our vaginas give off a squishy, squeaky sound. It's caused by air bubbles that get trapped inside of the vagina as you go in and out. It's normal and harmless, except it may embarrass her. Keeping her legs closer together or not coming out of the vagina too much can control it. Every position, angle, depth, or other variation will create a different sensation. Try everything at least once so you can create your CLB for total satisfaction for both of you. Add as much spice and variety as she likes. Don't forget to get into a steadier, consistent rhythm toward the end. Theresa said, "I want very slow intercourse at first, then faster."

 Hot Tip

Exercise together and then have sex. Cardio helps the blood flow to the penis, which results in stronger erections.

THE ANYTHING BUT ORDINARY MISSIONARY POSITION

The missionary position is a favorite for many of us. Almost every woman (and many of you) finds this the ultimate of intimacy. We can kiss, feel our breasts against your chest, connect through eye contact. Many of us love to end intercourse in missionary. You say you do too. Ted said, "There's nothing like feeling my wife's breasts against my body as I come." Emmet added, "I love kissing my lover during orgasm. It adds to my excitement."

However, women have a harder time coming in this position because you often don't make direct contact with our clit. So put your "clit radar" in place. A finger on her clit always feels good. Encourage her to finger herself. Lift your body higher on your partner and aim for the love button to stimulate it with each thrust. Try locating your pubic bone (the bone above your genitals) and get that into the act. When it hits the clit, hold your ears. Many of us say it's the best! Claire explained:

> I always liked intercourse but needed a hand or mouth to come. I assumed it was me. When I met Marc, intercourse became another experience. Every move hits my clitoris, sending me into ecstasy. I have many orgasms with Marc. I asked what he does. He said he raises his body just a bit so the base of his penis and anything near it hits my clitoris constantly. I see stars. I'm hooked on this man. Why don't all men do this? It seems so effortless for Marc and the results make sex much better.

Practice this technique. Men who do it say they get the same stimulation but more excitement—they know she's getting much more satisfied and that's a turn-on. Jesse said he drives us crazy with the "ten count" technique. He said it works especially well if your partner already had an orgasm and she's hot for your penis:

Rub the head of your cock around the clit and walls just inside. Then let just the tip go inside her about an inch and gently go in and out to a silent count of ten. Then shove it in—once. Then go back to the one inch in and out to a ten count. Then drive it home again—once. It'll drive her crazy the first couple of times. When she can't take it anymore, keep going.

Missionary works many ways. Your partner can lie with her legs flat or bring her knees up for deeper penetration. Use pillows underneath her for better angles. Her legs can be open or shut. Put her legs over each of your shoulders. Rub her clit when possible. Put both legs over one shoulder and then the other. That keeps her legs together. Sit upright on your knees and find other ways to move her. She can bend her knees to put her feet on your chest. Swivel her so she's lying on her side. Many of us love the change of positions, but stick with one way as orgasm gets closer. There are many ways to twist, turn, bend, etc. Just don't forget—*the clit is it!* Always aim to stimulate it whenever you can.

You on Bottom Smiling/Woman on Top

Many of us love being on top and many of you love the idea of us riding you while you watch. But some women aren't coordinated enough or don't have legs strong enough to bounce on you as much as we'd like. Being on top can take time for some of us to get used to. It can be hard on our knees. You may assume we all want it but not all of us are as anxious as you'd think. A majority of women can learn to love being on top though, because it offers us more control. And you can play with our breasts and clits, which is fun for both partners.

Keeping your penis inside us takes skill. If we bounce too high, whoops—or worse. You don't want us landing on your erect penis. Suggest she lean on your shoulders for support. That creates a good angle. If necessary, guide her. Keep your hands on her hips until she gets a good rhythm. Your partner should keep her body fairly close to yours, not rising more than a few inches. Try different ways. Rocking rather than bouncing works well in this position. The penis doesn't always have to go in and out a lot to stimulate.

If she keeps her body close to yours, it can prolong your orgasm because it's not as intense as other movements. Let her milk your penis, which means squeezing her vaginal muscles tightly against your penis, then letting go. Some of you say you love it. Women say it can intensify their pleasure. Make the most of her clit with your "clit radar." Many women say they love being on top because they're in control and can push their clit against you. Pull her forward so the base of your penis stimulates it with each movement. Position her so you can put as much pressure on the hot button with the pubic bone each time your bodies meet. If she's adventurous and wants to try hitting her G-spot, have her lean back, tilt her bottom up toward your face, and hold her hands as she rides your penis. Hold her steady. With the right angle, stimulation to her G-spot can make her explode with joy.

Another variety on top—have her face away from you. She can gently ease down on your penis and set her own rhythm. It's a good angle to control your body to nuzzle her clit for maximum stimulation. Hold her breasts as she rides you. Some women swear by this position to hit the G-spot for an intense orgasm.

For a different twist, sit on a chair with her on your lap facing you. Her body should straddle yours, penis inside, with her legs hanging down. It works better if her feet touch the ground from her perched position. This position offers the ultimate control, as Dee explained:

> Sitting on Don's lap on a straight chair is my favorite for orgasms. When I'm on top in bed I get tired—my knees hurt. On his lap I bounce using the full strength of my legs. I love total control. I can go as deep or shallow and as fast or as slow as I need, and love guiding my clitoris against his penis on each bounce. It's my instant orgasm position!

You can sit back and watch your partner bounce, play with her breasts, stimulate her clit, stop her a minute for a kiss, gently caress her all over, or lean back and enjoy her taking over your penis! She can also face the other way when she sits on your lap. That adds yet another delicious angle to add to your repertoire and her CLB.

DOGGIE STYLE

Do you think women like rear-entry intercourse? Those of us who've learned to appreciate it love to indulge. Yvonne loves the deep penetration and feels in total control. Paula enjoys being able to move back and forth on you. Some women don't like it because it lacks intimacy: the name isn't romantic; we may be self-conscious about you seeing our tush close up if we feel fat; we can't see you and don't feel connected since you're not holding us. But many of us cope because it feels so great! Kisses and squeezes help.

Since the name puts many of us off, refer to it as entering her from behind. It can make a big difference in her perception. "Doggie style" is unromantic. There are many variations for entering our vagina from behind. She can be on her knees with her upper body down or raised on elbows. She can lie flat on the bed. Sensations vary for each. Typical doggie is her on her knees. It's more comfortable if she props herself up in front with pillows and raise her tush high. If her head starts banging the wall or getting crunched because the movement pushes her forward, please stop a second and back her up!

Doggie style is fun—it allows for more vigorous thrusting and is the easiest position for us to thrust back in. It's the deepest penetration. Women who love it say you hit the G-spot often. Betty said, "Kneeling off the edge of a bed, behind in the air and being entered from behind as my lover stands on the floor gives great orgasms, especially for the G-spot." Some women enjoy lying on their stomachs, with you on top of them, pumping down like a jackhammer.

This is the easiest position for her to finger herself. Reach around and play with her breasts and clit. Theresa says it's her favorite position. "I feel it the most and can stimulate myself. I like my cheeks to be squeezed and rubbed from that angle." Because there's a lack of intimacy, your partner may prefer to end in the missionary position. Switch before your orgasm, if that makes her more receptive.

MORE INTERCOURSE SMILES

Spooning is holding each other while lying side to side in the same direction so that you and your partner fit together like two spoons. Lea said, "I can contribute better and with more control. When we're on our side, it's easiest for either my boyfriend or me to rub my clit. We don't have to balance and both hands are free." This provides most of the benefits of doggie style but it's more intimate. We love falling asleep in this position because of the intimacy and comfort it creates. Sex in this position can be slower and more sensual. Since you're both lying down, it's more relaxing and less rushed—a nice way to begin intercourse. Reach around and stimulate her breasts and clit while you're thrusting. Hold her while you're inside and caress all over.

A very intimate position is any variety of what I call Chillin' Inside. Prolong your orgasm by being inside without thrusting. She'll LOVE this. It's a great time for kissing and caressing and solidifies your connection. You can lie on top of each other, face each other sideways, or sit up with your legs wrapped around each other. Especially if you're with someone you love, this allows an incredible connection between lovers. Let her vaginal muscles squeeze your penis. Lie still or slowly move in circles. Stroke her face and hair, say nice things and be as romantic as you like. Kiss lots. We won't complain! Taking a Tantric sex class together can bring this to another level.

Try lying on your hip with your head propped in your hand. Your partner can do the same, facing you, and swing both of her legs over your raised hip in a way that your penis can slide inside of her. When you get used to this position, it can be a very comfy cozy way to chat—plan a romantic getaway or share poetry. There's easy access for massaging her clit, kissing, caressing, and loving looks. Don't do this if you're very horny and don't want to hold your orgasm. It's better after a round of sex. It's especially nice in the morning after a hot night of sex. You may be too tired for athletics but appreciate being inside her.

ANAL PLEASURES

A majority of you said anal sex appeals to you. A majority of women nixed it at the starting gate. Anal sex seems perverted to some of us. Many women were interested but said they probably wouldn't do it because it might hurt too much—your size would be a factor. We're also squeamish about having your penis in a place we see as unclean. Many women are horrified about you sticking your finger or penis in our tush and getting it dirty. Anal sex is an acquired taste. Those who love it say it's the ultimate sensation. Deep penetration reaches our G-spot from the best angle. The opening is much tighter than a vagina.

Approach your partner carefully about anal sex. It's a touchy request for many of us. When you're not having sex, explain why you'd like to try it. Perhaps have a book or information about the pleasures of anal sex to share with her. Don't pressure her to do it. If she's at least willing to consider it, begin with manual stimulation. Try a finger rubbing just inside her tush during oral sex or intercourse (sex shops sell little rubbers you can use on your finger). Women and men who've tried anal love beads (beads attached to a string that are inserted into the tush and pulled out quickly as an orgasm begins) say they intensify an orgasm a lot. Try an anal vibrator (one with stoppers so it can't go too far) with lots of lubricant. If she enjoys any of these she may be motivated to try anal intercourse.

A big problem for us, once we agree to your penis being in our tush, is anal sex can be painful. Sex stores sell butt plugs that stretch the opening gradually for those who are serious about anal play. Use lots of lubrication. You must use a condom for health reasons. Let her be in control if you get her to try it. Don't push yourself into her. Let her slowly back into you and set the rhythm. Be gentle in what you do. If she says it hurts too much, STOP! You may need to try several times before she relaxes enough. Or she may never want to do it again. Respect her choice. A word of caution: If you use a finger or penis anally, don't put it anywhere else until it's washed thoroughly, no matter how clean your partner is.

AFTERPLAY

After your orgasm, you may want sleep. You're known for insensitivity to our needs after active sex is over. Many of us don't feel sex is complete without reconnecting on an emotional level. That's what afterplay does for us. Delicious cuddling and caresses keep us happy. We see it as part of the sex act and like to feel that sex was more than a physical release. Ian said, "I offer them a warm washcloth, then clean them, then cuddle, kiss, and talk."

For some of us, this closeness afterward is our favorite part. The intimacy and "just-laid glow" are satisfying. We're more alert after sex, which is a fluke of nature since you may need to sleep. BUT DON'T JUST ROLL OVER AFTER SEX!!! Make an effort to sleepily kiss, hug, caress, and enjoy being wrapped up in the person you've just made love to.

I'm pleased that many of you acknowledge enjoying afterplay. But women still complain that some of you completely switch gears right after your orgasm. If you can't help falling asleep, let her know why when you're not in bed so she's prepared. When sex is over, we don't want to lose the connection it creates. Being held, cuddled, and kissed is important to us. In the morning we may try to keep you in bed or follow you around, touching. This holds our connection with you. We want to still feel one with you after sex. If you have sex during the day, take a catnap together. Then go for another round. A snuggling nap makes our connection strong and can build into part two.

 Sexy Tip

When you go to sleep, tenderly caress her leg, arm, or whatever is easy. It helps her feel connected as she falls asleep.

More Play

The possibilities are endless. There are lots of ways to keep the spice in your sex life. Here are some others that may help you. Be creative. Women consistently said their best lover was someone who communicated and made them feel comfortable sharing intimate desires and preferences. Give her lots of choices.

 Sexy Tip

Encourage her to wear a full skirt and leave her panties home.

SEX AT "OTHER" TIMES

You probably know that any time is the right time for sex. Many of us can't break out of the program that sex is supposed to happen after dark. Mornings can be lovely, especially on the weekend since there's no rush. But a quickie once in a while before work can be fun too. Your partner may not see the advantages of morning sex. Change her mind. On a scientific level, your testosterone levels are highest in the morning. Many of you wake up with a hard-on. On a practical level, you're already in bed. On a physical level, both of you are more rested than before going to sleep. Most of us feel more relaxed in the morning, unless we're late for work. On a healthy level, sex stimulates our bodies to secrete all sorts of hormones that are good for us and give us more energy—a great way to start the day! Keith said:

> I convinced Mindy we should set our alarm earlier at least once or twice a week. She balked at first. Now we both prefer getting up earlier to have sex in the morning. When we'd stay up later at night to do it, by morning we were regretting losing sleep when the alarm went off. Now the alarm wakes us up in anticipation so getting up earlier isn't hard at all. Mindy sees how relaxed she is at work, so now she sets the alarm.

Many of us don't feel attractive in the morning. We may have a hard time believing that with our hair messed up and no makeup we could look good. We may like having sex at night only—we can turn out the lights and you won't see what we perceive as our unattractive body. Let her know how much you're turned on seeing her by daylight, and how cute she is. If she feels her breath isn't perfect, get her some water. Or, before sex, have a quickie in the bathroom to brush teeth and use the toilet, which is healthier anyway.

You may hate to think much in the morning and don't want to do anything that can be construed as working. But romance can be easy and fun as you wake up. When you know she's rousing, start nibbling on her. It can be as simple as nips on her cheeks, shoulders, and neck, to going up and down her entire body. Rub your cheek gently on her breast, and if she responds, keep going. Gentle kisses are a delightful way to say "good morning." Start at her head and slowly work your way down her body. If she responds, go all the way down. Wake her up with your tongue in her vagina. Be careful about this if she may get upset. Once in a while, make a date for a whole day in bed! And many of us like surprises during the night too!

QUICKIES

Quickies are lots of fun, as long as you don't rely on them as your sole menu item. Quickie sex can also be quality sex. You need to get creative and find ways that quickly meets both you and your partner's needs. Ronnie said:

> My wife and I have hectic schedules. It's rare that we're both home at a reasonable hour. I had a hard time getting through the week without sex and suggested quickies. At first she was offended. Li said she wanted quality lovemaking, not just getting off. I did too—quick didn't mean skipping all the good stuff. She agreed to try. We let each other know what was most important to get satisfied. We actually start before going to sleep with kissing and caresses. In the morning we have some kisses and I go to her most sensitive areas, starting with oral sex. Li lets me know when she wants me inside of her. She's learned to have an orgasm, or at least enough pleasure, in a short period of time. She likes it a lot now. We both smile more at work and it's brought us closer, which she especially likes.

Quickies can be links in the ongoing connection we need. They give us more of the closeness we crave, as long as you don't skip tenderness. Quickies are especially good with a partner you've been with for a while. If you know her body well, you know how to make the most out of the time you have. Combine a morning shower and foreplay. Then hit the bed quickly and rinse off again before you leave for work. While you're doing other things, such as washing dishes, brushing teeth, talking on the phone, or working on the computer, use erotic gestures or rub each other seductively to turn each other on before you get to intercourse. Quickies shouldn't be one-sided. You both have to be passionate, horny, and dying for some quick relief and connection. Forcing a quickie on her isn't a good idea. Some of us feel degraded if you don't take the time to make love with all the trimmings. Show her how much fun they can be by giving lots of affection and making at least some time to please her too.

Quickies can be exciting. You might be alone somewhere and know it won't be for long and decide to make the most of those moments. If you have fifteen minutes before the repairman arrives, go for it. The pressure of time can intensify your desire. You can practice condensing the most intense aspects of sex into a brief but passionate liaison. Once she appreciates the pleasure they can bring, she can relax and enjoy more, reducing the time she needs to feel satisfied. Quickies in the morning can stimulate a need for more, which can make for great sex at night.

SEX IN ALL THE RIGHT PLACES

What's the right place for sex? Anywhere you choose! Although a bedroom is traditional, you can christen any room, floor, table, chair, etc. in your house. Be creative. Make her feel comfortable about breaking out of ruts. Close the shades and play music so neighbors don't hear her squeals. Go down on your partner in different locations. Put her on the kitchen table and eat her for breakfast. She can hang off the edge of a bed with you on the floor or sit on a couch or chair with you on your knees as you eat her. Armrests allow her to put up her legs for great access. Do you have privacy in your yard or pool? Figure out the rest!

Encourage your partner to try sex in different places. It's fun. Creativity keeps the heat in sex. She may be reluctant at first, so start with the most comfortable alternative. Throw pillows on the floor and do her there. Try the couch in the living room or the dining room table. A table or counter can be great for intercourse if the height is comfortable—great sex doesn't involve hurting yourself. If she wears a full skirt to go outdoors, you can get more adventurous. You can do a lot with the skirt as a shield. Your hand can stimulate her almost anywhere, especially in the car. Picnics can include her as dessert. Keep it playful. Getting out of the bed is fun and good for spontaneous sex.

Hot Tip

Spend a whole day together naked. Make a "no clothes" rule for the day.

If you have kids, roommates, or other people in your home, take advantage of times when you're alone. Send the kids to your parents for an overnight. If possible, play hooky for a day from work when everyone is out and romp around the house in ways you usually can't. You can let loose more if there's no one to hear you. Or, plan to go away for a night or two whenever you can. Make time to play! Remember my F & M (Fun and Money)? Don't forget to keep the "F" part active!

Edible Stimulation

Some couples use ice to enhance stimulation—everywhere. It can be rubbed all over your bodies as a contrast to the heat you're feeling. Rub an ice cube on her nipples before sucking them. Some of you keep ice in your mouth while sucking her nipples, clit, inner thighs, and other parts. But be careful—don't choke on the ice accidentally! Insert a small sliver of ice into her vagina right before intercourse for a cool sensation for both of you.

Lots of other edibles can be added to the blueprint. Whipped cream, chocolate syrup, marshmallow, beer, etc. can all taste good when licked off of various parts of your lover. Not everyone likes it but if you and your partners are munchers—indulge in a tasty feast. Edible flavored lotions can be added to the menu. Her CLB can include a large menu!

Accessories

If she doesn't get wet enough for a slippery entry, use a lubricant. Condoms can cause more friction than our natural lubricant can deal with so keep some on hand. A waterbased one is best. You can get K-Y Jelly in a drug store or more fun ones in a sex shop (or online). Lubricants come in different flavors and scents. They're nice to add spice during oral sex. There are all kinds of tasty accessories available (see Resources in Chapter 15).

I talked about vibrators earlier. They come in many varieties, shapes, sizes, and uses, in battery or electric. Small ones are handy when your hand or tongue gets tired. There are vibrators for the G-spot (curved in a way to hit the spot) and for anal use. Never use a vibrator in your tush that's not specifically made for it. It needs the stoppers at the bottom to keep it from going in too far. A small vibrator can work its way in deep if you let go of it. That's why they make special ones for anal stimulation. Check out the catalogues online. And don't forget, vibrators can give you pleasure too.

SEX DURING HER MENSTRUAL CYCLE

Are you turned off at the thought of having sex with your partner during her period? I don't recommend doing anything you're uncomfortable with, but a funny quirk of nature makes many of us hornier and more receptive to stimulation at this time of month. Some of us are too embarrassed to be turned on, but many of us would love sex if you didn't mind.

If you indulge, place a towel underneath. Test the waters if you're unsure. Set boundaries in advance. Most guys who've done it say that once they get aroused, little bothers them. If you just want to go with oral sex, she can leave a tampon in if she uses one. Take it out for intercourse! Jesse pointed out that blood doesn't flow from the clit so if you just use your tongue or finger on it, you can avoid it. Some of you who don't normally use a condom do use one at this time because you're squeamish about getting blood on your penis. Try it. You may love how responsive your partner can be.

~

You can have the hottest, most delectable sex possible if you want it. Expand your horizons, talk to your partner, try new things, develop confidence, and allow your feelings for her to motivate your lovemaking. Experiment until you have a very detailed and extensive CLB for your partner. Ian said, "Great sex starts with a great set of hands and tongue . . . spare nothing . . . get her to confess what she likes best. Let her know she is awesome and then prove it!" You can be her greatest lover. Repeat after me, guys—*the clit is it!* That's your key to great sex. Use it well!

15 *A Few Final Words*

W ell, my darlin's, we got through much together. I sincerely want you to have better, more satisfying relationships. We should all be on the same track—to please each other! Don't forget that you're not always easy to deal with either. You do things that can boggle our minds too! Men and women both have to bend to get along with each other. Let's! ~

I've given you the basics of how to satisfy a woman, in and out of bed. Now I'll emphasize some of the things I've said earlier and give you some final suggestions. They may work so well your partner may see you as the man of her dreams. You can thoroughly please a woman both in and out of bed if you choose to be flexible and give us some of what we crave. Work it! You'll love being with a satisfied woman who thinks you're the best thing that ever happened to her!

+ *Work with your partner.* A good relationship is teamwork. That means both of you. Never forget—you and your partner are on the same side. Don't let your program "to be simple" conflict too much with our complex nature. We can get along. Stay respectful in all interactions. And, maintain a good sense of humor—encourage her to do the same.

+ *Don't expect to get along all the time.* We all have good days and not-so-good days. Keep your expectations realistic. As long as you show each other respect and are willing to talk problems out using my Ten Commandments of Communication (see page 94 for a refresher), you can get through almost anything. Be straight with her. Don't keep anger in until you explode or do something dumb.

+ *Maintain your connections.* A kiss; hug; tender touch; "wonderful to see you"; a note—it's those little things that make a big difference. Don't take them, or her, for granted. Creating connections keeps the sparks warm. And sparks are easier to ignite than cold stones, both in and out of bed! Keep them warm and you'll maintain your passion for each other.

+ *Make time for each other.* Quality time creates the foundation of a very satisfying relationship for both of you. Give her your undivided attention regularly. Find time to talk every day. Let her know how much she means to you. Make love to each other as much out of bed as you do in it. All the delicious menu items in Chapter 12 enhance your relationship.

+ *Make friendship a priority.* As the relationship grows, never stop nurturing the friendship between you. That means making sure to let her know she's appreciated. Do whatever you can to develop trust between you. Verbally share experiences with her. Have goofy times. Make sure little things like cooking together are kept fun. It makes chores more pleasant. Don't let the passing of time allow you grow apart.

+ *Enjoy sex as one facet of your relationship.* If you want to be in a healthy relationship, let sex be the icing on your already delicious cake! Enjoy it as an activity for sharing a joyous experience with your partner and enhancing your relationship. Don't forget that sex is supposed to be fun! Think of it as play. Don't take yourself too seriously during sex. Learn to laugh with your partner.

+ *Make time for sex.* While sex shouldn't be the most important thing between you, regular sex is healthy. Talk to your partner about making it a priority. Tell her how much it means to make love to HER regularly. Make dates to have an intimate evening on a regular basis. Look forward to it. Let her know your anticipation earlier—include HER in the excitement, not just the act. Call during the day or leave her a note at home or in her briefcase—"Can't wait to be with you later!"—"I love you and am looking forward to loving you tonight!"—"Think of what I'll do to you tonight and get as aroused as I already am." What you say, of course, depends on your partner. Some women enjoy a more explicit note than others.

+ *Make time for intimacy.* Even when time is scarce, you're tired, or not quite in the mood, give her tenderness and fore-play. If you may not be able to get it up, level with her. You can make love tenderly without an erection. Sometimes you may get one when you least expect it! Even if you don't, pleasure her with your hands and mouth. She can please you too. Love-making doesn't require an orgasm. If you can put aside your need to achieve, you may find making love without an orgasm a very delicious activity that brings you closer together.

+ *Don't use sex as a tool to get your way.* Using sex to manipu-late your partner or as a substitute for treating her well in other areas won't allow the most loving intimacy possible. We feel used. Women complain about men who are warm and loving in bed and cold and inconsiderate out of it. We're not responsive after a while with men like that. Don't be one.

+ *Don't use sex to solve problems.* Some of you prefer to make love instead of dealing with problems. That doesn't help a relationship. We may smile a bit before the next fight, but not for long. Sex isn't an antidote for anything but horni-ness. Yes, tender lovemaking may appease us when we're upset with you. Yes, tension is relieved temporarily with sex, putting problems aside for a while. Sexual intimacy brings us closer momentarily, but it won't solve problems. Difficul-ties with communication, anger, unfair expectations, and other angst-provoking situations won't get fixed under the sheets. Using sex to keep a relationship from falling apart just prolongs bad feelings. Even if we're happy during sex, what bothers us doesn't go away. It will surface after your orgasm. Talk out of bed first!

Using Your New Tools

Well, you sweet, delicious opposites of my sex, it's time for you to pack your toolboxes and use them to build a happier, more satis-fying relationship for you and the woman you're with, or keep them handy until you meet a healthy one. I've provided you with a kinder perspective for accepting and working with the curve balls and dif-ferent agendas that my soft, fun, and delectable sisters often hit you with. Please understand I made many generalizations that must be tailored specifically for your partner.

I used to be a stereotypical female. Thanks to my dad I had more autonomy than most women, but my self-esteem was still con-tingent on you. I believed my life was nothing without a guy and was never truly happy. I did a lot of Daylle-bashing and drove many of you crazy. Three factors changed me. One, I faced that I wasn't happy with my life, even when I had a boyfriend. Two, I realized that guys had a right to be who they are and it was my choice to go/not go along with what didn't suit me. Understanding where your different programs come from enabled me to get along with you much better. And three, I began saying "I love you" in the mirror, even though I didn't feel it. Eventually I stopped seeing myself in the distorted mir-ror that told me I was fat and unattractive.

As my self-esteem and self-love grew, I didn't just accept the dif-ferent ways you approach life. I now rejoice in them. I really love you guys and have learned from you! Today I'm thrilled with me as I am. For the first time in my life I feel ready to be in a healthy rela-tionship. My faith is strong that the Universe will guide me to the right partner. It really does work! Since I faced many of the demons that women have, I have great compassion for those who still strug-gle. It can be painful, especially when guys make us feel worse by trivializing or mocking our needs. They can be difficult to deal with.

Honestly, many women get on my nerves too! Switching into compassion mode makes a big difference.

I implore you to develop compassion. That may be hard for some of you but it's well worth the effort. Compassion is a virtue that's well rewarded. It tempers the anger that our actions and needs can stimulate. Understanding our needs enables you to make us feel better, without a big effort. When your partner has needs, she's not your enemy trying to hurt you. Make her happy as you would your friend.

I'll leave you with a bit more mushy stuff. Love yourselves. Appreciate the essence of who you are and don't change it for a woman. Work on creating a sense of faith in a higher being to help you get through trying times. I wouldn't be where I am today without it. Faith is the backbone of my existence. Develop your confidence based on the healthy aspects of who you are. Grow as a man by facing your feelings and learning to compromise in your communication. Get therapy if you need it to sort out old stuff. If you find the *right* therapist, your life can open up to marvelous treats!

I wrote this book because I sincerely want *both* sexes to be happy. Unless you plan on giving up women, allow your attitude toward us to change. And don't forget—say something nice to her (and mean it) every day, appreciate her and make her feel special, strengthen your patience when she acts insecure, maintain your connections, don't take your partner for granted, love yourself, don't let past fears keep you from present joys, and *the clit is it!* You go, guys!

Resources

Alexander Institute: A source of adult videos, including ones that are designed for instruction.
Web site: *www.lovingsex.com.*

Condomania: Another source of condoms and lubes.
Web site: *www.condomania.com* or 800-9-CONDOMS.

Condoms 4 Free: This web site, *www.condoms4free.com,* allows you to try different brands of condoms.

Good Vibrations/The Sensuality Library: A source of sex toys, vibrators, and adult videos.
Phone: 800-289-8423. Web site: *www.goodvibes.com*

SafeSense: A source of a good assortment of condoms and lubricants in flavors and textures.
Web site: *www.safesense.com*

Sinclair Institute: A source of adult videos, including ones that are designed for instruction. The site also has sex toys, adult videos and more.
Web site: *www.bettersex.com* or call 800-955-0888.

Daylle Deanna Schwartz is always gathering information and welcomes your input. She would like to hear from both men and women about your positive steps forward and personal experiences that you learned from. She would also like to hear from anyone who would like to be interviewed or who would fill out a questionnaire for her future books. Your anonymity is guaranteed. ❧

Contact Daylle Deanna Schwartz at:
daylle@daylle.com
www.daylle.com

Printed in the United States
By Bookmasters